Heal Yourself with

TRADITIONAL CHINESE MEDICINE

Find Relief from Chronic Pain, Stress, Hormonal Issues and More with Natural Practices and Ancient Knowledge

Dr. Lily Choi, L.Ac, D.Ac *and* Bess Koutroumanis

PAGE STREET
PUBLISHING CO.

First published in 2023 by

Page Street Publishing Co.

27 Congress Street, Suite 1511

Salem, MA 01970

www.pagestreetpublishing.com

Distributed by Macmillan, sales in Canada by The Canadian Manda Group.

27 26 25 24 23   2 3 4 5

ISBN-13: 978-1-64567-748-2

ISBN-10: 1-64567-748-6

Library of Congress Control Number: 2022945425

Cover and book design by Meg Baskis for Page Street Publishing Co.

Photography by Madeleine Kilgerman. Dr. Lily's author photo by Flora Hanitijo. Graphics by Bess Koutroumanis.

Printed and bound in the United States

Dedication

I'd like to dedicate this book to my father for opening the door to

Traditional Chinese Medicine and to mother for carrying out the

principles of Traditional Chinese Medicine in our daily life.

CONTENTS

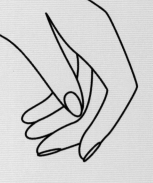

PART 2:

TREATING ILLNESSES, CONDITIONS AND HEALTH ISSUES 56

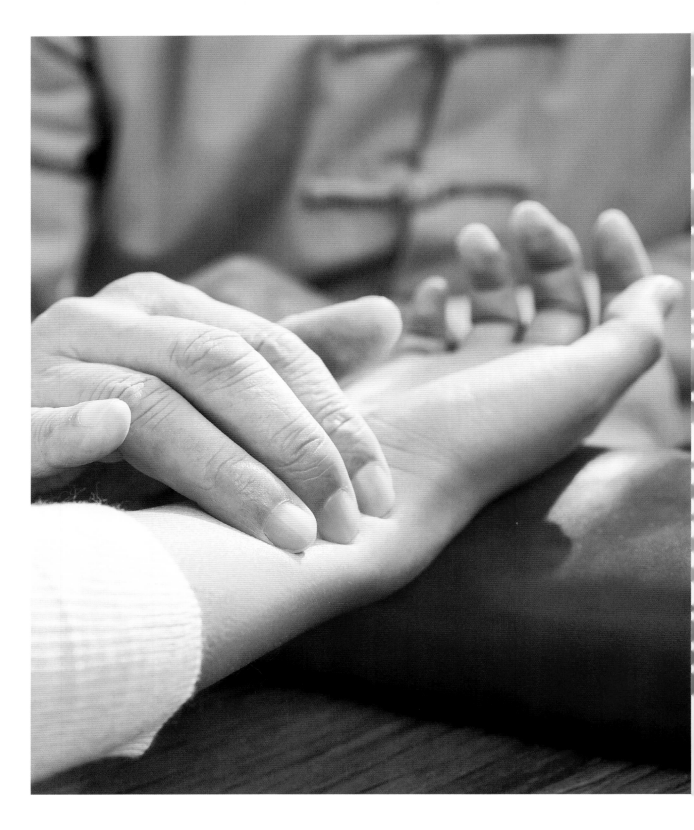

Introduction

Dr. Lily Choi

After the unexpected passing of my father, I was determined to keep my mother around for as long as possible. Although I always had an interest in natural medicine because my dad was an herbalist and owned an apothecary, it wasn't until I experienced the feeling of his loss that I felt my purpose.

I began studying books on medicine and eventually began attending school for it. I had an interest in both modern and ancient practices. I realized that many of the basic principles of Traditional Chinese Medicine (TCM) were instilled in my daily life by my mom. The most common examples are that she wouldn't allow my siblings and me to leave the house in the morning without having congee (more on that later), with wet hair or without dressing warmly. We always ate home-cooked meals, had medicinal broths and our plates changed with the seasons.

My parents lived this lifestyle and these simple, yet influential habits poured into my life. More than that, my mom was always happy and joyous. That was the most influential thing she passed on to me that I will never forget. My upbringing gave me more of a clear direction. I continued on with my studies and became a certified acupuncturist and a doctor of Chinese medicine. I was able to apply my learnings to my mom as I had hoped and kept her vibrant and healthy for all her 96 years.

My philosophy is if you love your body, respect nature and have a positive outlook, you will live a happy and healthy life of longevity and vitality.

Bess Koutroumanis

In my early twenties, I went through a near-death experience. The way I had been living wasn't representative of who I was and the path to that realization was a challenging one.

On operating tables and in and out of the intensive care unit, I was told by my doctors that my survival was nothing short of a miracle. I was lucky to be alive. After a slow and arduous recovery, I was given the green light to resume regular life. In this transition, although I was assuming normal life, I was far from feeling as though I was. I began to develop autoimmune conditions and was left with many symptoms that were interrupting my daily life.

All I could think was "Wasn't I supposed to be getting better?" I felt helpless and defeated. At this point, I felt like I had used up all the strength I had in this lifetime. Although I felt extraordinary gratitude for my life, something just felt off. I longed to feel vital once again. Watching all my friends and peers living their lives was hard while I was constantly fatigued, sick to my stomach, suffering from anxiety and migraines, post-traumatic stress disorder and Crohn's disease. One day, I reached my threshold. I knew there had to be another way.

At the time, I wasn't aware of "alternative" medicine or holistic treatments, but the protocol I was on felt like a Band-Aid approach that was simultaneously creating new problems. I began researching acupuncturists in my area and came across Lily's practice. I set up an appointment and, from the moment I walked into her practice and met her, I immediately felt like I was able to exhale the deepest sigh of relief. I had opened a door to new possibilities and the helpless feeling that I had almost surrendered to ceased. It is miraculous what the body does with just a little hope. This hope rang through my body like a bell signifying a new beginning.

The rest, as they say, is history. Learning to treat my symptoms with TCM has changed my life and, eventually, got me off all medication. It added value in all areas of my life, especially my emotional and mental health. Being treated and eventually mentored by Lily has been one of the biggest blessings in my life. She truly embodies all the wisdom and medicine she teaches, and I believe that's why so many people are positively affected by her practice and even just through her presence.

What I'd like to say is if there is a more seamless path for you to self-discovery, health and awareness, take it. Don't ignore the signs—honor your mind, body and spirit. As my Qigong Master, Grand Master Nan Lu, says, "The body never lies."

What You Will Gain from This Book

Optimal health. We all want it, but very few of us know how to achieve it.

Traditional Chinese Medicine (TCM) is a practice that originated in ancient China. Although it has been molded and has taken shape over the centuries, the guiding principles have stayed the same. These look different from the Western ideals you may be used to. Through this book, you will learn these principles and reexplore your health through this ancient lens. You will learn to nourish your emotional and physical health with new forms of healing, such as acupressure, herbs and meditation. Above all, this book will show you the connection between you and everything around you. If you feel like you've been plagued by ailments, illnesses, and mental and emotional funks, and Western practices didn't help, this book is for you.

All healing is self-healing, which means *you have the power*. Learning basic methods of TCM can connect you to the self-healing ability that exists within you. To realize this capacity, you must connect to all the aspects that make you who you are. Imagine you have three bodies: the mental, the physical and the emotional. All three of these entities make up the synergistic whole of who you are. You can't live without any of them; they are the three seeds that bloom to create you. Each part must be tended to, watered and fertilized to grow beautifully. In this book, we will begin to break this concept down, understand it and heal with it.

Part 1

THE FOUNDATIONS OF TRADITIONAL CHINESE MEDICINE

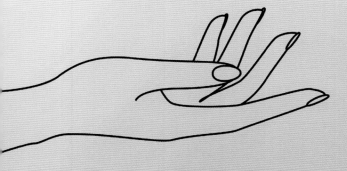

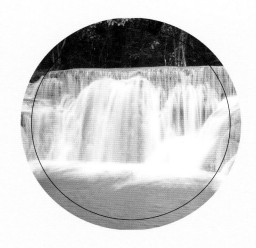

Chapter 1

The Basic Principles of Traditional Chinese Medicine

Before we start exploring how to heal ourselves with TCM, we need to understand the guiding principles of this practice that form together into one beautiful orchestration of harmony. In this chapter, we'll explore a brief history of this ancient tradition and go over some key foundational schools of thought. This will help you get familiar with the lens through which TCM practitioners view the body, health and the world. Although it may feel like a totally new way of looking at things, I promise it will start to make sense as all the pieces of the puzzle come together. Keep these principles in the back of your mind when we think about healing in the chapters to come.

A Brief History

TCM is a healing system that dates back between 2,500 and 5,000 years ago and has changed very little since its conception. It is rooted in Taoism's credence (or Daoism) on the human connection to nature. *Tao* literally translates to "the way" or "the path." In accordance with the Tao, TCM believes that well-being is achieved when one lives in harmony with nature and, therefore, with natural law. Natural law is universal, applying to everyone, everywhere, in the same way, whether you are aware of it or not. This theme was understood thousands of years ago and again in modern physics.

This ancient medicine was developed by the sages and masters who were said to have summoned this wisdom during their meditative practices. TCM was birthed through spiritual practice, and those very doctors contributed greatly to the arts, literature, dance, sculpture, calligraphy, painting and to poetry especially, which they used to further convey their knowledge of medicine in a concentrated, yet deeply moving way. Each phrase about the body in TCM held a picture to portray the union of the body with the emotion and spirit.

> *"The harmony of natural law reveals an intelligence of such superiority that, compared with it, all the systematic thinking and acting of human beings is an utterly insignificant reflection."*
>
> —Albert Einstein

Written sometime between 2600 BC and 300 BC, the most important ancient book of Chinese medicine, *The Yellow Emperor's Classic of Internal Medicine* (黄帝内经), is still considered the doctrine of TCM.[1] This book takes the form of a discussion between the famous Chinese emperor Huangdi and his physician, in which Huangdi inquires about the nature of health, disease and treatment.

The Yellow Emperor's Classic of Internal Medicine departs from old shamanistic beliefs about disease and focuses on disease as a byproduct of diet, emotions, lifestyle and environment. This text introduced the concepts of the universe being made up of the principles of Yin and Yang, Qi and five phases or elements (these are all concepts we'll explore further in the pages to come). It details how these forces work harmoniously with one another and everything around them. Health is a manifestation of that harmony and balance of these natural forces. Humans are seen as a microcosm that mirrors the larger macrocosm. All forces that apply to the universe apply to humans.

How can this esoteric intelligence help us in our modern society? It is deemed standard in today's world to suffer from things like anxiety, migraines, stomach discomfort, hair loss, and menstrual pain and irregularities (all of which we will dive into, by the way), but what if I told you that these symptoms are not, in fact, normal? In TCM, these are signs of body dysfunction and an alert that there is a deeper imbalance within. These symptoms are warning signs, sent out in hopes of preventing a more serious condition in the future.

---

1   Curran James, "The Yellow Emperor's Classic of Internal Medicine," *British Medical Journal* 336, no. 7647 (2008): 777, 10.1136/bmj.39527.472303.4E

"We but mirror the world. All the tendencies present in the outer world are to be found in the world of our body. If we could change ourselves, the tendencies in the world would also change. As a man changes his own nature, so does the attitude of the world change towards him. This is the divine mystery supreme. A wonderful thing it is and the source of our happiness. We need not wait to see what others do."

—Mahatma Gandhi

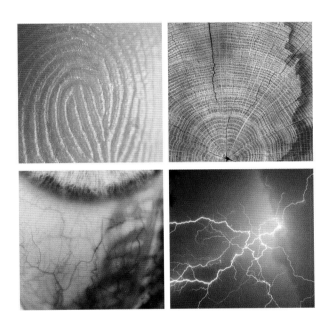

We Are Mini Universes

So, how are we so related to nature? Our body is made up of the same basic elements that make up the earth. There is a universal force that generates and moves everything in it. Humans are part of this force and are themselves mini universes, guided by the same forces that guide our larger universe. That is why we look at nature for guidance, support and as a mirror to our mini universe inside.

The body is made up of complete and highly sophisticated interconnected systems just as the universe is. If one part of your body or mind needs attention, you'll likely heal other parts of yourself as well. And when humans are doing the work to truly heal themselves, it creates a synergy with the environment. A world of healthy people is quite different from a world of sick people.

We live in nature and nature lives within us.

The Root Cause Effect (Root vs. Branch Approach)

One of the core principles of healing with TCM is the root versus branch approach. This can be viewed best by an example. Let's use acid reflux (we go over this condition in depth on page 58), which is the result of stomach acid flowing into the esophagus or throat, causing burning sensations in the chest. The most common treatment for this is to take any one of the many medications available to eliminate the symptoms. Antacids, which are regularly prescribed for acid reflux, block the production of acid.

This approach is not addressing *why* the body is creating the excess acid, but instead it covers up the effect of how the body responds to it. This is exactly what we refer to as a branch treatment. It provides temporary relief but does not create a chance for the problem to stop occurring. It's like pruning branches of a diseased tree but not looking in the soil to find out why the branches are coming up sick.

The branches are the visible manifestations of the problem, while the roots are what is going on deeper in the organ systems of the body. Only trimming and cleaning up the damaged branches won't help when the roots are sick. The branches will keep growing back, diseased. The root cause treatment, however, would be to find out why the body is creating the excess acid and why it is flowing upward. Treatments for the root cause would be to uncover any physiological disturbances and address them to heal the actual problem and to stop it from occurring.

The branch treatment usually relies on medication to address the symptom. This offers temporary relief, but the symptom is likely to reappear. If you use the branch treatment long enough, you also must consider what side effects any medication will cause. For every action, there is a reaction. Each and every thing we ingest on a physical, a mental and an emotional level requires assimilation by the body.

The root cause or root treatment approach aims to target the underlying imbalance creating the symptom. This way takes more time and requires patience and consistency, but it can ultimately show results and create a more resilient body. While the branch approach uses medication to get immediate relief, the root solution makes your body stronger so that you are resistant to those things recurring.

"The superior doctor prevents sickness, the mediocre doctor attends to impending sickness, the inferior doctor treats actual sickness."

—Famous Chinese proverb

Prevention Is the Best Medicine

In TCM, the goal is not only to correct illness but to prevent it from happening. We are always understanding and nurturing our bodies to prevent against symptoms, diseases and fast aging so we can lead a better quality of life. I recently spoke to an older patient of mine who said, "If I'd known I was going to live this long, I'd have taken better care of myself!"

We can think of this with a metaphor: Every durable house begins with a strong foundation. If there are any cracks in the foundation, it must be tended to for the structure to remain safe and stable. The taller the house, the stronger the foundation must be to live harmoniously within its natural environment and withstand natural elements. A taller house gets you a better view. For your healthy life, the higher you can build, the better you will feel. When you build a strong foundation, your potential can reach the sky! You can build a beautiful life with a clear perspective and unobstructed views of your dreams.

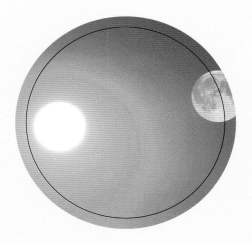

Chapter 2

Understanding the Body Through Traditional Chinese Medicine

When you begin to view your body through the lens of TCM, you will start to see your body in a different light—one in terms of striving for balance. You'll understand how to use your energy to create harmony. Imagine your body is made up of a series of gas tanks and you can see where you have fuel and where you need it. You could then decide how far to go depending on how much fuel you have! Through the lens of TCM, you will be much gentler on your being and appreciate it even more. These virtues can support your healing process in a very deep way.

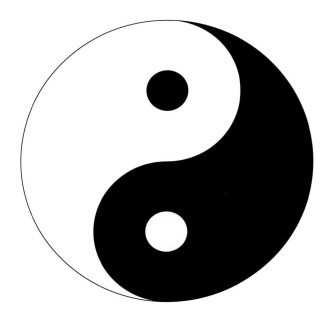

"The law of Yin and Yang is the natural order of the universe, the foundation of all things, mother of all changes, the root of life and death."

—The Yellow Emperor's Classic of Internal Medicine

The symbol shows that Yin and Yang forces cannot exist without each other; they are inseparable and constantly becoming one another. Each half contains a small circle in the center of the opposite color. This reveals that each side carries the essence of the other. The curved line that separates the two showcases that, although they are opposites, there is no definite separation. Together they form oneness, the way day flows into night and vice versa. Yin and Yang are in a constant dynamic dance with each other. This dance denotes that all things affect one another, as everything, all things, exist together.

So, how does this all relate to TCM and your health? In TCM, disease is diagnosed and treated based on the balance of Yin and Yang.

The dual energies of Yin and Yang must always work in harmony. If there is too much of one energy, there will be too little of the other, which creates an imbalance. Imbalances will show up as problems in the organ systems manifesting as symptoms and illness.

Yin and Yang

The Yin-Yang symbol is recognized all around the world. It was first referenced around 700 BC in the *I Ching (Book of Changes 易經)* and since then has influenced almost every aspect of Chinese culture, including martial arts, science, politics, traditions, feng shui and more. It serves as the guiding principle of TCM, its very own North Star. This symbol is the foundation of diagnosing illness and understanding wellness.

The philosophy of Yin and Yang states that all phenomena are composed of two opposite but mutually interconnected forces known as Yin and Yang. This duality is not just about opposites; to merely view it as such would be too simplistic. The duality encompasses the transformation, balance and harmony within us and outside of us in our material world and in nature.

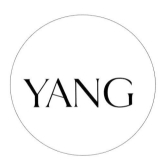

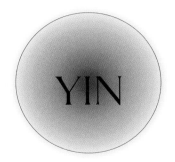

YANG	YIN
Masculine	Feminine
White	Black
Light	Shade
Day	Night
Sun	Moon
Fire	Water
Heat	Cold
Dry	Wet
Spring & Summer	Autumn & Winter
Hard	Soft
Active	Calm
Fast	Slow

What Is Yang?

"陽者，若天與日，失其所，則折壽而不彰" translates to "Yang is like sky or heaven and like day and sun. When it is lost, life is broken, shortened and disease and sickness arrive."

The Yang (陽) character means masculine, sun and bright.

Yang is the transformative, creative force of energy that activates and warms the body. When Yang is sufficient in a person, they feel energized as Qi (energy; we'll do a deeper dive into the concept of Qi soon) is flowing freely and all bodily functions are effectively performed. For example, when Yang is sufficient, Qi moves normally in the abdomen to move toxins through the intestines, allowing the body to digest adequately, transform food to nutrients and detox waste.

If Yang is deficient, there is less power for action! Since Yang creates movement and normal bodily functions like digestion rely on movement, they become less efficient, which negatively impacts the entire body. That is why when Yang starts to dim, so does the quality of life.

Yang deficiency is a term you will hear a lot about in TCM and in this book. When we refer to deficiency in general, it is emphasizing that something is weak and has a lack of energy or vitality.

Yang deficiency results from many habits that are quite common. The most frequent habits I see are over-consuming cold foods and drinks, overexertion and exceeding your body's threshold without proper recovery, skipping breakfast, chronic stress, constant information overload, overexposure to cold without proper precaution, lack of proper sleep and imbalanced emotions.

- **Symptoms of Yang Deficiency:** body pain, weight gain, thyroid problems, liver disease, stomach disorders, kidney disease, infertility, menstrual imbalances, cysts, cancers and tumors.

How Can We Nourish Our Yang Energy?

- **Through Foods:** Spices such as ginger, cinnamon and nutmeg; animal proteins, Bone Broth (page 121) and eggs; grains like rice; chives, scallions, leeks, mustard greens, pumpkin, longan fruit and lychee all contain a "warming" energy, which acts like a match to ignite the fire needed for action.
- **Through Lifestyle:** Balancing rest with assertiveness, exercise and work. Go to bed early and rise with the sun. Receive sun on the body, especially on the back. Have regular meals and don't skip breakfast or lunch and eat lighter at night. Avoid exposing the belly region around the umbilical cord and the back, as cold easily penetrates and weakens life force from this area. Always wear slippers and socks when on cold floors.

What Is Yin?

The character for Yin (陰) means feminine, moon and cloudy.

Yin is the energy that grounds us and helps us accept what is in order to balance the active nature of Yang.

Yin is the fluid that is used to moisten our body, specifically all the organs, cells, Blood vessels and glands. Blood is considered a Yin fluid (we talk more about the important role Blood plays in TCM on page 23). If we lack Yin, all our body parts can easily become rigid, become overheated and lose proper function. Yin energy is responsible for the moistening and cooling of bodily functions. It is also associated with the feminine because the menstrual cycle typically lasts 28 days, like the moon cycle.

When this energy is depleted, your body begins to show signs of "heating up." This is not a true heat but rather an artificial one, signaling that your internal thermostat needs some maintenance. Moistening and cooling functions are necessary to maintain a healthy balance in temperature, bodily functions and overall stability.

Yin deficiency results from excess output without enough stillness or restoration.

- **Symptoms of Yin Deficiency:** hot flashes, fatigue, night sweats, vaginal dryness, lower back soreness, general discomfort or weakness, dizziness, occasional ear ringing, dry skin, unquenchable thirst, irritability, insomnia, easily angered or frustrated, nocturnal emissions, sore throat, chronic swelling of gums and chronic toothaches.

How Can We Nourish Our Yin Energy?

• **Through Foods:** Eat vegetables like avocados, artichokes, asparagus, green leafy vegetables, wild yam and zucchini; fruits like apples, mulberries and persimmons; proteins like adzuki beans, black beans and tofu. Avoid spicy foods and alcohol.

• **Through Lifestyle:** Practice daily meditation, go to bed before 10:30 p.m. and perform moderate exercise without too much perspiration.

Maintaining the Balance of Yin and Yang

Yin and Yang are always striving for harmony with one another in response to one's experiences. In its most simplistic form, as mentioned earlier, disease or dysfunction is a result of the imbalance of Yin and Yang—when the mutual restraint of the opposite force becomes out of control. This creates either an excess or a deficiency. Each organ system has their own levels of Yin and Yang, as each system makes up smaller parts of a whole.

1. **Yang Deficiency**
2. **Yin Deficiency**
3. **Balanced**
4. **Yin and Yang Deficiency**

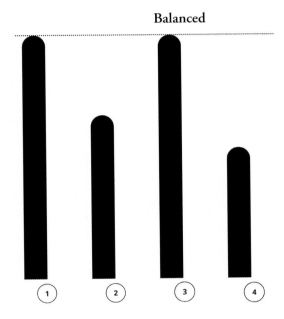

The Three Treasures: Jing, Shen and Qi (and Blood)

The *three treasures* determine your physical, mental and emotional health. *Jing* relates to the physical structure of your body, *Shen* to the part of you that is self-conscious and *Qi* to the active processes created by and involved in regulating the relationship between these two.

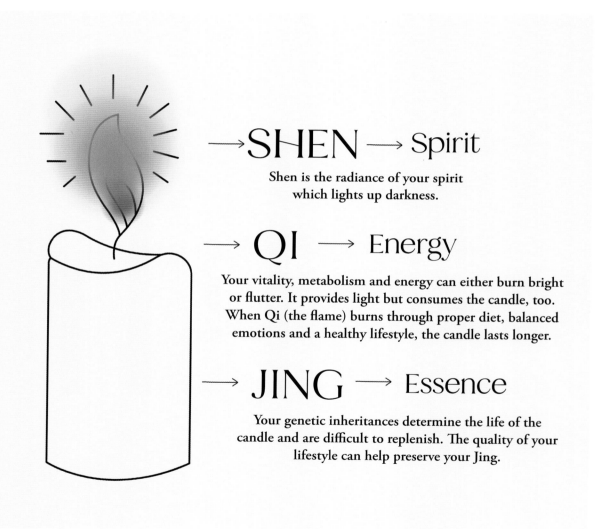

→ SHEN → Spirit

Shen is the radiance of your spirit which lights up darkness.

→ QI → Energy

Your vitality, metabolism and energy can either burn bright or flutter. It provides light but consumes the candle, too. When Qi (the flame) burns through proper diet, balanced emotions and a healthy lifestyle, the candle lasts longer.

→ JING → Essence

Your genetic inheritances determine the life of the candle and are difficult to replenish. The quality of your lifestyle can help preserve your Jing.

Jing — Our Essence

Jing translates to "essence," which we inherit at our conception. Although there is no exact translation of Jing, it is similar to our DNA, as it's inherited from birth, is the carrier of your heritage and makes you who you are. The Chinese character for Jing (精) indicates a substance that is derived from a process of refinement and purification, implying that this material is one to be cherished and protected.

"Essence" is the organic substance that forms the basis of growth, reproduction and development. The term is used in three ways in TCM: pre-heaven (prenatal) essence, post-heaven (postnatal) essence and vital essence. Prenatal essence is inherited from our parents and can't be replaced. Postnatal essence is produced by the Spleen from the food we consume so it can be nourished. And vital essence is what we call Jing and it is stored in the Kidneys. Therefore, there is a naturally close bond between Jing and the Kidney system.

Jing powers the battery that provides us the energy to perform our life functions and circulates through the Eight Extraordinary Meridians (page 44) to create bone marrow, menstrual blood and semen. The natural decline of Jing during our lifetime leads to the natural decline of sexual energy and fertility as we age.

The more you nourish your postnatal Jing, the longer you will keep your prenatal Jing and the healthier you'll be. If you lead a life of moderation and balance, you will keep a good amount of your reserve Jing energy saved up in your savings account. If over the years you take too many withdrawals, you may start to encounter problems associated with aging much earlier.

WHAT DEPLETES JING?

- Overexertion in all forms: mental, physical and emotional
- Chronic stress
- Staying up late and insufficient rest
- Alcohol and drug abuse
- Excessive ejaculation and excessive sexual activity

HOW TO NOURISH JING

- A healthy digestive system
- Working through emotional trauma, barriers, patterns and issues
- Cultivating a meditation, Qigong or Tai Chi practice
- Receiving acupuncture and practicing acupressure to support energy flow in the meridians
- Eating eggs, animal proteins, organ meats, Bone Broth (page 121), bee pollen, kidney beans, sea vegetables, royal jelly, black rice, black wood ear mushrooms, walnuts and black sesame seeds

"The body is to nature as a violin is to an orchestra. The strings are to a violin as the organs are to the body. For the orchestra to play in harmony, all the instruments must be tuned to each other. If a single instrument is out of tune, the whole sound is dissonance rather than harmony."

—Between Heaven and Earth: A Guide to Chinese Medicine

Shen — Our Spirit and Mind

Jing and Qi have a close relationship. Together, they are believed to form the foundation for Shen.

The term "Shen" is frequently translated as our "spirit," but it encompasses one of the most complex concepts of TCM. Traditionally, the term refers to the mechanism of change, the mystery of sudden and profound transformation and the expression in a person's face, particularly the eyes. When applied to the human body, the term describes a major part of what would be called physical vitality, mental activity and spirit.

Shen is loosely translated to our spirit and mind, which is housed in the Heart. It refers to the part of us that is spiritual but is not about our beliefs. Rather, it focuses on our consciousness, emotions and thought. Shen is said to preside over activities that take place on the mental, spiritual and creative planes.

The spirit can be harmed by external factors if we fail to maintain vitality through good habits, physical strength and adequate nourishment. The spirit can also be harmed by internal factors, especially excessive emotions.

When the Shen is healthy, you will have clear thoughts and be rational. You will generally feel calm and peaceful and have healthy relationships. A disturbed Shen manifests as poor concentration, memory loss, irritability, anxiety, insomnia and other signs of mental and emotional disorders.

I hope that you are beginning to see the correlation of our mental, emotional and physical health being one system—and how each one impacts one another greatly.

Qi — Our Energy

Qi, pronounced "chee," is the vital force of all living things. It is the very substance that sustains us and allows the body to perform all of its physiological functions. Qi contains aspects of both energy and matter. Throughout the book, we will refer to it as energy, knowing very well that energy and matter transform into one another.

How cool is it that modern physics and Eastern philosophy are very much aligned? $E = MC^2$. It's the world's most famous equation by Albert Einstein that states "Energy equals mass times the speed of light squared." On the most basic level, the equation says that energy and mass (matter) are interchangeable; they are different forms of the same thing. A person's vitality is a manifestation of their Qi. Whatever manifests within a person does so because of their Qi—it can describe every aspect of life.

Although Qi is a broad subject, we can categorize it into two main buckets: an inherited Qi and a cultivated Qi. We inherit Qi from birth, which acts as our energy savings account, which is the type that can't be replenished. The type of Qi that can be cultivated is derived from the food we eat, transformed by the Spleen and Stomach system, and from the air we breathe, transformed by the Lung system (more about those systems to come). The healthier those organ systems are, the more efficient both the quality and quantity of Qi that is formed. Qi is considered a Yang substance because of its active nature.

Blood

Blood is a larger concept in TCM than we know it to be in Western medicine. Blood is not just the same blood that comes out of a cut; it is also an energy force that flows through the body delivering warmth, moisture and nourishment. It is considered a Yin substance and nourishes and moistens our entire body. It also supplies the basis for our mental activities. Although Blood is not one of the "three treasures," without it we would be without Qi—they are inseparable energies that need one another. Qi and Blood are not the same but they are inseparable and interdependent; Blood is considered a dense form of Qi. When Qi moves, Blood follows.

The primary functions of Blood are to provide nutrients for organs, tissues and our meridians (more on page 42); maintain healthy body movement and sensations; and support a healthy mind and mental activities.

Blood deficiency is the most common imbalance experienced with Blood, as it manifests into many types of physical, mental and emotional issues.

- **Symptoms of Blood Deficiency:** pale and dull skin, particularly in the face; dry and pale lips; weak muscles or muscle spasms; dry skin; blurred vision; poor memory; insomnia; tingling, numbness or cold extremities; dizziness; hair loss or premature grays; fatigue; lighter and shorter periods; anemia; and limb weakness.

HOW DO WE BUILD BLOOD?

When I speak about building Blood, I mean nourishing and promoting healthy levels of it. The primary way to support Blood is through our diet because the digestive system supports its production.

If the food source is red or dark in color, chances are it tonifies the Blood. Animal proteins (especially grass-fed red meat and beef liver), Bone Broth (page 121), dark leafy greens, cruciferous vegetables, root vegetables, black and kidney beans, beets, avocados, blackberries, raspberries, goji berries, Chinese red dates, cherries and pomegranates are all great food sources for tonifying Blood.

As a general guideline, foods rich in iron, vitamins B12 and C, folic acid and protein are great for Blood-building. Foods like dark leafy greens contain chlorophyll, which is very similar to hemoglobin, but instead of iron at the center, it has magnesium.

All the recipes outlined in Chapter 6 (page 113) are able to build the Blood!

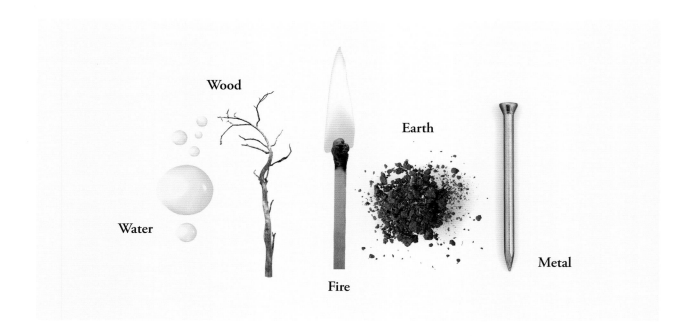

Wood

Earth

Water

Fire

Metal

Five-Element Framework

The Five Elements reflect a deep understanding of natural law, the universal order underlying all things in our world. The ancient framework denotes the Five Elements, or five phases of life: Wood, Fire, Earth, Metal and Water. Each of these natural elements are associated with different organs in the body, colors, flavors, senses, emotions, weather, sounds, direction—so on and so forth—to create a range of interconnectedness and unique relationships between the internal and external worlds. It also emphasizes the importance of the dynamic balance among the organ systems of the Liver, Heart, Spleen, Lung and Kidney. The whole body is completely connected with its own communication system through multidimensional relationships. Health comes from a harmonious balance of all the elements.

Although the organs have the same names as they do in Western medicine, their meanings differ. In TCM, the organs are a larger concept than just anatomical structures. That's why you see organs capitalized in this book, to reference their greater meaning. These systems represent broad and intricate networks that contain channels of life force weaving in and out of each other, yet still occupying separate territories.

An organ is considered for its physiological and psychological meaning. In TCM, the internal organs encompass aspects of the emotions, mind and spirit.

Five-Element Framework

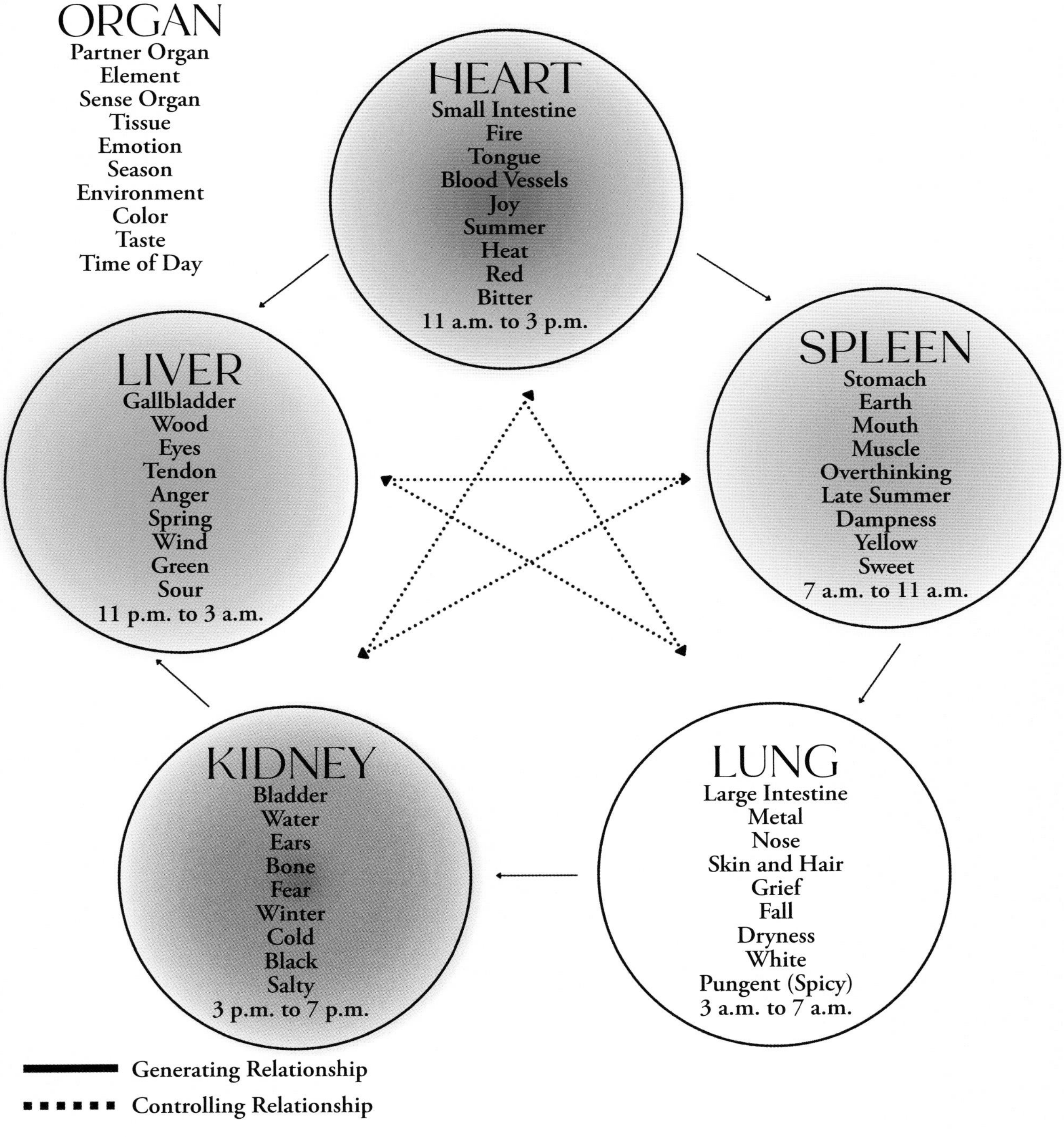

ORGAN
Partner Organ
Element
Sense Organ
Tissue
Emotion
Season
Environment
Color
Taste
Time of Day

HEART
Small Intestine
Fire
Tongue
Blood Vessels
Joy
Summer
Heat
Red
Bitter
11 a.m. to 3 p.m.

SPLEEN
Stomach
Earth
Mouth
Muscle
Overthinking
Late Summer
Dampness
Yellow
Sweet
7 a.m. to 11 a.m.

LIVER
Gallbladder
Wood
Eyes
Tendon
Anger
Spring
Wind
Green
Sour
11 p.m. to 3 a.m.

KIDNEY
Bladder
Water
Ears
Bone
Fear
Winter
Cold
Black
Salty
3 p.m. to 7 p.m.

LUNG
Large Intestine
Metal
Nose
Skin and Hair
Grief
Fall
Dryness
White
Pungent (Spicy)
3 a.m. to 7 a.m.

—— Generating Relationship
■ ■ ■ ■ ■ Controlling Relationship

How Do Organs Relate to Each Other?

Zang (臟) and Fu (腑) are the two types of internal organs. One complete pair is made up of one Yin organ and one Yang organ to partner together to create one balanced system.

- **Zang organs are considered Yin.** They are solid and store essence. They are the Liver, Heart, Spleen, Lung and Kidney.
- **Fu organs are considered Yang.** They are hollow and receive and transport. They are the Gallbladder, Small Intestine, Stomach, Large Intestine and Urinary Bladder.

By nature, Yang organs are always rotating between filling and emptying actions. They are usually empty cavities, transmitting nutrients to the body with a connection to the outside and play a role in digestion. Just as the Yin-Yang symbol indicates, one cannot exist without the other: A Yang organ must be partnered with a Yin organ. Yin organs house vital substances like Blood, Qi, Yin and Yang. Each organ relies on it its partner to function for optimal health.

Since everything is connected, this five-element framework shows us how each individual system reacts with one another. The two types of lines on the chart on page 25 showcase two different types of relationships with great significance. The *Generating Relationship* is the solid black line and is best compared to the relationship between a mother and child. A mother provides energy to fortify the growth and health of her child, as part of the health of the child relies on being nourished by the mother. The *Controlling Relationship* is the dashed line and represents a relationship that can act as a restrictive energy or an attacking force. Without proper control, things could fall out of proportion. These relationships act like a checks and balances system.

The Liver System

Partnered Organ: Gallbladder

In the modern person, the Liver is the most affected organ system. Stimulants, chemicals, environmental toxins, processed foods, excessive unhealthy fats and life's daily stressors have left this essential organ system as congested as a freeway at rush hour. This is essential to pay attention to because, in TCM, we need a healthy Liver to live a healthy life.

The Liver is viewed as the commanding general of the body. The general's duty is to protect and defend its troops and countrymen. The Liver protects, defends and commands the 500 plus tasks it does for the body on a daily basis.

The main responsibilities of the Liver are the regulation of emotion, the promotion of digestion and absorption, and the maintenance of smooth circulation of Qi, Blood and body fluids. It also supports reproductive function. The Liver is also the most important organ in relation to women's health. It stores Blood, regulating the volume during physical activity, rest and during menstruation. Hormonal balance and cholesterol are governed by the Liver.

"The physician who knows how to harmonize the liver knows how to treat the hundred diseases."

—Du Yi Suibi (Reflections Upon Reading the Medical Classics)

The Liver System

Element: Wood

Sense Organ: Eyes

Tissue: Tendons

Emotion: Anger

Season: Spring

Environmental Factor: Wind

Color: Green

Taste: Sour

Time of Day Liver: 1 a.m. to 3 a.m.

Time of Day Gallbladder:
11 p.m. to 1 a.m.

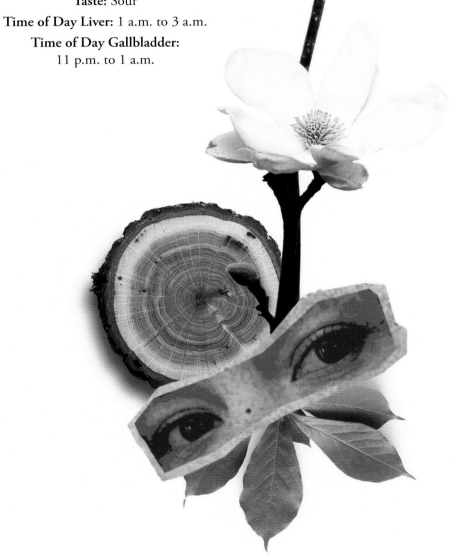

Wood, the element of the Liver system, requires flexibility physically so it does not break. Similarly, the Liver—with its flowing energies that require upward and outward distribution like a tree—requires flexibility to bend so it does not break. Wood burns to create fire, just like the fire we require to fuel our digestion, which the Liver promotes.

When Qi, Blood and emotions are flowing freely, one is happy and content. Those with harmonious Liver systems are calm, fluid to life's ebbs and flows, have strong decision-making skills and a clear vision. When this flow is blocked, symptoms arise. Many factors can create stagnation, like our environment, foods and lifestyle, but, most of all, our emotions are the leading cause for stagnation of the Liver system.

The eyes are the sense organs of the Liver. The Liver opens to the eyes and moistens them. Tears are considered the fluid of the Liver. Crying is healing for the Liver system because it takes the invisible (emotions) and turns them into the visible (tears), expressing and releasing stored energy.

The tendons, the tissue of the Liver, are controlled by the Liver, as it is responsible for mobilizing the Blood that moistens and nourishes them.

Spring is the season of the Liver system and it is a time that blesses us with new beginnings. The energy is expansive and surging forth, pushing up through the hibernation of winter and signaling renewal and rebirth.

When the Liver system is experiencing dysfunction, one may have pain, dizziness, anger, depression, eye problems, irritable bowel syndrome symptoms, brittle nails, springtime allergies, headaches, irritability, indecisiveness and fluctuation of mental states.

Gallbladder

The Gallbladder is considered a Fu (hollow) organ. But unlike its other Fu counterparts, it does not transport impure waste. Instead, it stores bile, a pure fluid. Like Zang organs, such as the Heart, it cannot be accessed through an exterior entry to the body. This makes the Gallbladder an "extraordinary organ" for its unique properties.

In the emotional body, the Gallbladder holds the need for respect and the ability to make decisions. It is the organ that has the courage to act on the plans of the Liver and create turning points for new beginnings in life. It is responsible for decision-making, judgment and courage. It also has a close relationship with the Heart. The Gallbladder's decisiveness helps the Heart control the mind. It helps guide the Shen and provides direction for it. Just as spring is a birth, the Gallbladder is a pivot, a turning point for new beginnings and new stages of life.

Even if you've had your Gallbladder removed, you still have your Gallbladder meridian, which is a channel of energy relating to the Gallbladder. This channel can be stimulated with acupressure, acupuncture, gua sha and Qigong.

Symptoms That Signal Imbalanced Liver Energy

Gallbladder: stones, removal

Eyes: dry, itchy, red

Tendons: stiffness, decreased mobility

Anger: easily angered, irritable, frustrated

Sour: cravings for sour taste

Time: experiencing nightmares, excessive dreaming and/or waking up between the hours of 11 p.m. and 3 a.m. when the Liver and Gallbladder are most active

Key Takeaways on the Liver System

• Eat lots of green foods! Green is the associated color of the Liver and spring. Focus on lots of greens and sprouts and cook them lightly rather than eating them raw (page 117).

• Stretching helps the tendons and sinews, and helps the flow of Qi and Blood throughout the meridians.

• The Liver has a great influence on creativity and expression, so express yourself through whatever creative medium resonates with you: painting, dancing, writing, sculpting, music or gardening.

• Liver energy is more involved with planning while the Gallbladder is for taking action. Spring is a great time to set goals because of the energy of renewal, but don't forget to take action with your new goals so that you don't feel stuck.

• Let go of constantly wanting to be in control. Change is the only constant in life and, when we practice being more fluid than rigid, we are less angry, irritable and stressed, all emotions that disrupt Liver flow.

• Goji and schisandra are berries that are classified as Liver herb super-healers.

• Since these organs are most active during 11 p.m. and 3 a.m., it is best to be asleep so the system can focus on detox and repair.

"The heart is the ruler of the five organ networks. It commands the movements of the four extremities, it circulates the Qi and the Blood, it roams the realms of the material and the immaterial, and it is in tune with the gateways of every action. Therefore, coveting to govern the flow of energy on earth without possessing a heart would be like aspiring to tune gongs and drums without ears, or like trying to read a piece of fancy literature without eyes."

—Huainanzi (Contemplations by the Huainan Masters)

The Heart System

Partnered Organ: Small Intestine

The Heart is the king of the body, coordinating all physical, mental, emotional and spiritual activity. The Heart is the seat of consciousness and intelligence, the master of Blood and the commander of the vessels. The Heart is the home of our Shen, dispatching it to the other organs. The Shen requires the Blood to keep it in place and the health of the Shen depends on the health of the Heart and Blood and vice versa. It all comes back to balance.

Shen plays an important role in our sleep: All insomnia issues (page 93) are said to have a root in Heart imbalance. The Heart is the house of the Shen. If the Heart is disturbed, the Shen has no residence and will wander around at night, causing sleep issues like disturbed sleep, excessive dreaming and an inability to fall asleep.

Fire is the associated element of the Heart. Fire gives life and light. When our mind, body and spirit are working harmoniously, we are clear. Think about a time when you've felt like you can accomplish anything! Your Heart was balanced and supporting you.

The tongue is the sense organ related to the Heart. When people talk incessantly, talk very quickly or laugh inappropriately, therein lies disharmony. Speech has always been held in the highest regard for many traditions around the world. Words are the truth of the Heart because they exhibit the connection between Heart and mind. The tongue also denotes taste, so not being able to taste food very well can also indicate an imbalance in the Heart system.

Perspiration is the "fluid" of the Heart. Spontaneous sweating means the energy (Qi) of the Heart is weak (what we often call a Heart Qi deficiency).

It is especially important to note the Heart's relationship with its generating and controlling organ systems (noted on the Five-Element Framework graphic [page 25]). The Spleen organ system is generated from the Heart. As mentioned, this is like a mother and child relationship. If the Spleen (child) is happy, the Heart (mother) is content. Good digestion equates to a healthy Heart. Additionally, the Liver generates the Heart. When Liver energy becomes compromised, say due to high stress, and is unable to regulate emotions, it is imbalanced and unsupportive of the Heart.

The Heart System

Element: Fire

Sense Organ: Tongue

Tissue: Blood vessels

Emotion: Joy

Season: Summer

Environmental Factor: Heat

Color: Red

Taste: Bitter

Time of Day Heart: 11 a.m. to 1 p.m.

Time of Day Small Intestine: 1 p.m. to 3 p.m.

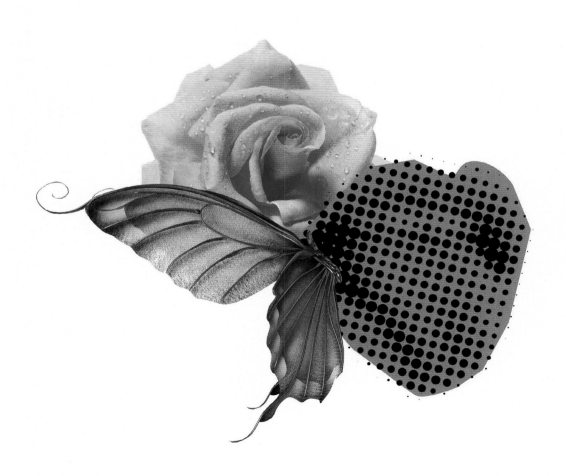

Small Intestine

The Small Intestine receives food and fluids from the Stomach after the Spleen has extracted their valuable essences. The Small Intestine is quite mighty, as it processes what the Stomach was not able to, but it is very affected by the temperature of food eaten. Continuous consumption of cold drinks and cold foods such as salads make this organ cold and unable to sift through waste properly. In TCM, cold is a pathogen taken very seriously (we talk more about that on page 47). It constricts and stagnates, disrupting flow.

The Small Intestine system controls the way we receive and absorb both food and information. It separates the "pure" from the "impure" by working with the Bladder and Large Intestine. Just as it does for foods and liquids, the Small Intestine plays a mental role, separating clear thoughts from the murky ones, therefore relating greatly to the Heart and mind.

Symptoms That Signal Imbalanced Heart Energy

Small Intestine: abdominal pain

Tongue: dry and dark red, tip may be red and swollen

Blood Vessels: pulse may be feeble and irregular if Heart Qi is weak

Joy: overexcitement to the point where you become out of control

Bitter: can have a bitter taste in the mouth

Time: symptoms like palpitations or shortness of breath could signal an imbalance in the Heart if it occurs between 11 a.m. and 1 p.m., and if you experience bloating, gas or vomiting between 1 and 3 p.m., it could signal an imbalance of the Small Intestine. Furthermore, if you haven't drank enough water during the day, you are more likely to feel dehydrated during this time.

Key Takeaways on the Heart System

• Many red foods benefit Heart function and even come into season in the summer. Eat foods like watermelon, cherries, tomatoes, red apples, beets, radishes, rhubarb, red lentils, longan fruit, red dates, chilies, red beans, berries, saffron and beef.

• Hawthorn is a berry used as an herbal treatment that nourishes the entire body, but, specifically, it has healing properties for the Heart because it is used to invigorate the Blood, treat hypertension and heart disease, and reduce body fat.

• We can strengthen the Heart by consciously and gracefully speaking our mind, living our truth, showing care and compassion, connecting to nature and experiencing joy.

• Meditation offers deep relaxation and observation of who we are. Through the mind, we ultimately can take care of the Heart, as they are directly linked. Practice a healthy mindset.

• San Qi (page 135) is an herb used to improve circulation and regenerate red Blood cells.

The Spleen System

Partnered Organ: Stomach

Learning about this organ system, you'll realize the deeply interdependent relationship between the body and mind. Once this connection is realized, you can live more intentionally, as the health of one relies on the other. More and more modern research is shining a light on the connection between the mind and gut, something recognized in TCM since its conception.

"病從脾胃生" This ancient TCM saying reveals that "all disease originates in the Spleen and Stomach."

Our Spleen is the source of Qi, Blood and bodily fluids. Along with its partner, the Stomach, this organ system oversees digestion, absorption and the transformation of food into nutrients that are transported out to the entire body, supplying our energy and creating Blood. Along with the Liver and Heart, this system is responsible for the production of the quality and quantity of Blood; it also helps support circulation. Just as Mother Earth nurtures everything on this planet, the Qi formed in the Spleen nourishes each and every crevice of our entire being.

"The stomach is called the sea of grain and water; everything is assimilated here. The spleen is in charge of transportation; everything is moved by its workings. Absorbing and moving: These are the essential actions which define the spleen/stomach network as the main source of the life-sustaining postnatal energy."

—*Gu Jin Yitong Zhengmai Quanshu (The Compendium of Traditional Diagnosis)*

Because they are our digestive organs—and our body and minds are connected—they are responsible for everything we take in, which includes everything we see and think. Just as they digest our food, they digest our thoughts and feelings. This is another connection to the mind.

Like the earth's soil, the digestive organs thrive on conditions of warmth and moisture. The temperature of the Stomach and Spleen is about 98.6°F (37°C). When cold substances are ingested, the Stomach first needs to warm it up, pulling Qi and heat upward from the lower body to help. Immediately, there is a decrease in circulation, which results in cold below the waist. This all takes place even before digestion. Liquids, including water, are digested just as food is.

Our Spleen governs our mouth, its affiliated sense organ, and lips, in addition to overseeing fluid metabolism. So, manifestations of weak muscles and dry and cracked lips are a sign that there are issues with fluid metabolism in the digestive system.

Muscle tone becomes a concern during the aging process, so much so that skin treatments, procedures and Botox® are at an all-time high. Did you know that a strong Spleen system results in strong muscle tone, especially in the face? The muscles are the tissue associated with the Spleen, and the Stomach meridian runs through the face (more on meridians on page 42).

Late summer is considered a season in TCM. It begins around the third week of August until the autumnal equinox. During this time, nature is experiencing its last bit of expansion time before harvest. Just as nature does, it is a compelling time of self-nurturing and self-cultivation, supplying us with transformative energy. Just as Mother Earth supplies nature with sustenance, our digestive system supports us emotionally, as well as physically.

The Spleen System

Element: Earth

Sense Organ: Mouth

Tissue: Muscle

Emotion: Overthinking

Season: Late summer

Environmental Factor: Dampness

Color: Yellow

Taste: Sweet

Time of Day Spleen: 9 a.m. to 11 a.m.

Time of Day Stomach: 7 a.m. to 9 a.m.

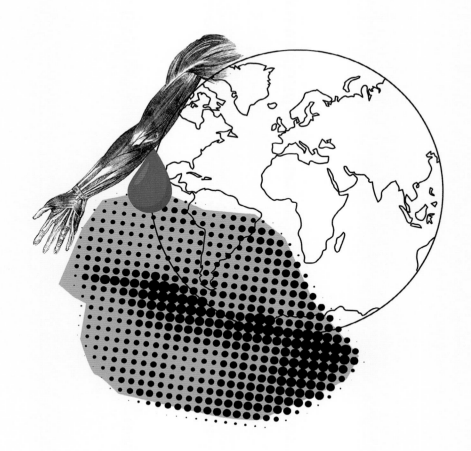

Stomach

The Qi flow of the Stomach is essential for carrying out the difficult task of digestion, as it is responsible for transforming the food and drink we ingest. Healthy Stomach Qi always flows downward, as this is how food should continue to move after it is processed by the Stomach. If there is an imbalance, the flow of Qi is either stagnant or in the wrong direction, leading to unpleasant digestive symptoms.

"Rotting and ripening" is the process of fermentation, which prepares the way for the Spleen to extract the refined essence from food. After this extraction takes place, the Stomach moves the remainder to the Small Intestine for further filtration and absorption.

Symptoms That Signal Imbalanced Spleen Energy

Stomach: nausea, no appetite in the morning

Mouth: dry or cracked lips

Muscle: weak muscle tone, muscle stiffness

Overthinking: excessive feelings of worry and anxiety

Sweet: cravings for sugars and sweets

Time: feeling nauseous in the morning or having no appetite for breakfast can signal weak Spleen system energy

Key Takeaways on the Spleen System

• Digestive organs love warmth. They love to be warm and love to be fed warming foods both in temperature and essence. Foods like ginger, sweet potatoes, rice, root vegetables, peppercorns and cinnamon are staples in TCM for their digestive power.

• Warm and hot drinks have a positive effect on your systemic cooling mechanisms and truly hydrate you.

• Ginger is the most beloved food of this organ system as it is warming, grown in the soil and has a yellow hue.

• Overthinking and worry are the emotions related to the Earth element. Focus on the now and what you can control. Work on healthy boundaries and learn how to graciously say "no" so you don't over-extend yourself.

• Spend time in nature, as that will be the best way to refuel, recharge and reconnect. Grounding is especially important for those with digestive issues and gardening is especially therapeutic.

• The Spleen ingests not only food, but every single bit of information that comes into the body through our sense organs. Currently, it is the norm to be connected and available 24/7, receiving information through texts, emails, news and calls. Have you ever felt like you needed a moment to process something you read or heard? That is because, just like food, we need to break down information into understandable quantities to process it. Be conscious of what you choose to digest: How you feed your mind correlates to your health and happiness.

• Have dinner by 7 p.m. at the absolute latest to give your digestion and other organs like the Liver time to rest. You will boost energy and get rid of excess weight this way.

• Positive emotions of the Spleen are fairness, openness and trust.

• The Spleen and the Stomach are most active between 7 and 11 a.m. They require fuel in the morning (breakfast) to perform their tasks. Skipping breakfast leads to weak digestive function.

The Lung System

Partnered Organ: Large Intestine

Just as a metal object absorbs the temperature of its environment in an instant, the metal organ system, the Lung, and its partner, the Large Intestine, are most easily affected by external influences. The Lungs are positioned at the upmost part of the body among the five organs and act as a delicate canopy, bridging the connection of our external and internal environment. They are our first line of defense from external pathogens.

The primary function of the Lungs is to manage the air and water within the body and, most importantly, regulate the flow of Qi.

"Wei Qi" is a type of Qi that is translated to our immune system and acts as a first line of defense. It is very much influenced by the Lung system. In order to protect the body, the Lungs disperse this defensive Qi all along the body's surface in order to warm it. If the Lung Qi is weak, the Wei Qi will be as well, resulting in a lower ability to protect the body and a weaker immune system.

External conditions like environmental cold, heat and dryness or internal dryness of the Lung or Large Intestine all have the potential to injure the fluid supply of the body. This can cause dryness symptoms in the nose, throat, Lungs, skin, body hair or intestines. In addition to being easily harmed by dryness, it passes on the condition as a symptom, which is why dry hair can be a direct result of an imbalanced Lung system.

Our boundary to the world begins with our skin (the tissue of the Lung system), so, for ultimate Lung function, we also want to respect the boundaries we set for ourselves as well.

Grief, sadness and melancholy are the emotions associated with the Lung system. If one indulges in these emotional states in an excess amount or for an extended period of time, harm to the Lung network will result and symptoms of lack of energy or dry skin may occur.

The Spleen system generates the Lung system; therefore, a well-functioning digestive system is vital for healthy Lung function.

Large Intestine

The Large Intestine and Lung duo is associated with beginnings and endings. According to *The Yellow Emperor's Classic of Internal Medicine*, the Large Intestine "transports all turbidity. All waste products go through it."

At first, the Lung paired with the Large Intestine may seem odd, but after uncovering these organ functions, it makes perfect sense. The Lungs breathe in oxygen from the air and breathe out carbon dioxide, the waste product of respiration. The Large Intestine also gets rid of waste from the digestive process. Also related to this partnership is the skin, another detox organ. All these organs remove what is no longer useful and create space for the new. These organs can cleanse the body, mind and spirit when they are harmonious.

Many times, when someone complains about consistent sinus issues and imbalances, I ask about their bowel movements. In most cases, their bowel movements (Large Intestine) are compromised, affecting the sinuses (Lung).

The Lung System

Element: Metal

Sense Organ: Nose

Tissue: Skin and hair

Emotion: Grief

Season: Fall

Environmental Factor: Dryness

Color: White

Taste: Pungent (spicy)

Time of Day Lung: 3 a.m. to 5 a.m.

Time of Day Large Intestine: 5 a.m. to 7 a.m.

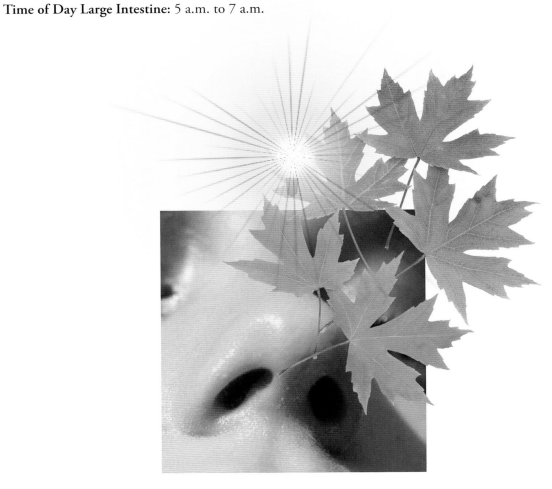

Symptoms That Signal Imbalanced Lung Energy

Large Intestine: constipation

Nose: congestion, runny nose, sneezing, loss of smell

Skin and hair: skin issues, dry hair

Grief: melancholy and sadness, feelings of grief

Pungent: cravings for spicy foods

Time: consistently waking up between 3 and 5 a.m., which could signal an imbalance and is common with those dealing with unresolved grief

Key Takeaways of the Lung System

• White foods nourish the Lung like garlic, scallions and daikon, and pungent foods such as onions, garlic, turnips, ginger and horseradish help to disperse mucus.

• Apples and pears nourish and moisten Lung fluids, particularly when poached or steamed. Try this during fall to combat dryness.

• Take time to tidy up the physical world around you and let go of what you no longer need. Clean the overlooked areas of your home, as this signifies a breath of fresh air.

• Astragalus (page 130) is superb in strengthening and toning energy and the immune system.

• Fall is the season of harvesting and collecting. We move away from the expansiveness of summer and start to prepare for winter. To do so, we must become more internal and introspective.

• Catching colds frequently is a sign of weakened Wei Qi and Lung Qi.

• The specific time for the Large Intestine is between 5 and 7 a.m. It is best to wake up and empty the bowels during this time.

The Kidney System

Partnered Organ: Urinary Bladder

The Kidney system consists of the Kidneys, Urinary Bladder and adrenals. This system regulates the body fluids and the excretion of wastes via the urine and is responsible for the tears, saliva, perspiration and the fluids that lubricate the joints. It is vital for the function of all the organs and tissues in the body and has the largest influence on the ears and bones.

In TCM, the Kidneys are known as the root of life. This system is responsible for storing our deepest levels of energy, our life essence Jing (page 20) and everything responsible for our growth, maturation and reproduction.

"In relation to the other organ networks, the kidney is situated in the lowest position. It is associated with the phase element water, and it is in charge of storing essence (jing). Just like water was the first substance to emerge from heavenly oneness, the kidney is the source of the human body, the initial sprout of physical life."

—Tushu Bian (A Compendium of Illustrated Texts)

When organs are running short on energy, they rely on the Kidney system to supplement their energy. That is why symptoms of premature aging like early gray hair, joint pain, bone issues, dental problems, hearing troubles and sexual dysfunction are all treated through the Kidneys. When we burn our energy too hard and too fast, the Kidney suffers.

The Kidney System

Element: Water

Sense Organ: Ears

Tissue: Bone

Emotion: Fear

Season: Winter

Environmental Factor: Cold

Color: Black

Taste: Salty

Time of Day Kidney: 5 p.m. to 7 p.m.

Time of Day Urinary Bladder: 3 p.m. to 5 p.m.

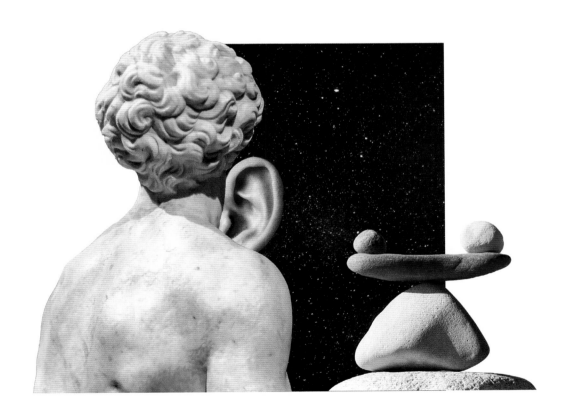

When the Kidney system is balanced you will have healthy fluid regulation and the skin, joints and sexual organs will be moist, hydrated and pain free. You will feel energized, lively with vitality and have strong bones, teeth, hearing and a healthy libido. Our Kidneys support the healthy transition through the different stages of life.

Our Kidneys also manage our stress response. When the body is stressed, the adrenals use up potassium and sodium to manage the stress by secreting stress hormones. Have you ever noticed that people who experience major stress look like they have aged more quickly? That is no coincidence.

In wintertime, the season correlated to Kidney energy, we are asked to be the most Yin (page 16) by becoming still and introspective. If we look at nature, it shows us the way. Fall is a time to let go of any excess we cannot carry—like the shedding of leaves—and in winter the trees become bare, which results in palpable quietness. It is time to go within. We tend to go against nature's wishes and push ourselves especially around the time of the holidays, resulting in lower immunity as the new year approaches. Going forward, think of your energy as your life force. When any situation or event arises, ask yourself, "Do I want to spend my Qi on that?"

Water is the element of the Kidney system. Out of all the elements, Water is the most destructive. Our very survival is threatened equally by its lack and excess. On an emotional scale, when the Water element and Kidney system are imbalanced, our mind and spirit can feel flooded or eroded, creating a fearful home for the body. We may feel completely depleted like our reservoirs are empty and we are scared.

Urinary Bladder

The Bladder's main function is to excrete water from the body through urine along with the ureters and urethra, which form our body's very clever filtration system. It serves as a reservoir of water and a filtration system all in one. The waste is secreted using Qi, the vital life energy, and heat energy from its partner, the Kidney. The urinary system is also responsible for electrolyte balance and hormone production, and it plays a part in the maintenance of healthy Blood pressure.

The organ partnership provides much support to one another. If there is a weakness in the Kidney functioning, it can be treated through the Bladder meridian, which runs on either side of the spine and down the length of the back (read more about this channel on page 44). One example of this is when people experience back pain, which almost everyone does at one point in their lives. Because the Kidney governs the back and knees, it can easily be treated through the Bladder meridian, which runs through the back and down the back of the legs.

Symptoms That Signal Imbalanced Kidney Energy

Urinary Bladder: frequent urination or urination issues

Ears: deafness, tinnitus, ear infections

Bone: osteoporosis, dental issues, joint pain, lower back or knee pain, developmental issues

Fear: severe panic attacks, anxiety, fear

Salty: cravings for salty foods

Time: If you crave sugar from 3 to 7 p.m., or feel as though you need a boost from caffeine, it could signal a Kidney imbalance because the Kidneys regulate our overall energy. It can also signal that you haven't eaten wisely enough before this time to create stable blood sugar.

Key Takeaways of the Kidney System

• Tap your teeth! The teeth are considered the "surplus" of the bone. Through daily stimulation, you can help your energy, aging symptoms and the health of your teeth and bones by tapping your teeth. Practice for 1 to 3 minutes, twice daily. You can even do it for 30 seconds at different points in the day, to add up to 1 to 3 minutes.

• Use acupressure on your ears to help increase Kidney energy. Rub them for 5 minutes every day. Stomp your feet, slowly and with flat feet, for about 5 minutes a day to stimulate Kidney energy. Kidney and Bladder meridians run through the heel and to the sole of the foot.

• Food that is cooked low and slow—like porridges, stews and soups—support the Kidney.

• Animal proteins like lamb, organ meats and bone marrow are especially helpful to build Kidney energy. Bone Broth (page 121) is important to consume, as the Kidney loves salty flavor and is connected to bones.

• Salty-essence foods and foods grown in the water such as wild fish, sardines, oysters and seaweed nourish the Kidney because they are associated with the water element and taste salty.

• Black-colored foods like black sesame seeds (page 76), blackberries, mulberries (page 134), black rice and black wood ear mushrooms are especially healing for this organ system.

• Beans—black, kidney and adzuki beans—are Kidney-shaped, resembling seeds and showcasing the potential for new life, just as our Kidneys govern reproduction and growth.

• Walnuts specifically tonify the Kidney system, strengthen and increase Kidney Qi and Jing, and treat pain and weakness in the knees and back that stem from Kidney imbalance. Walnuts help with Kidney deficiency, impotency, sexual dysfunction, infertility, frequent urination, back and leg pain, and stones in the urinary tract. Toast them for a few minutes to make them even more digestible before consumption.

• 3 to 7 p.m. is for great mental concentration.

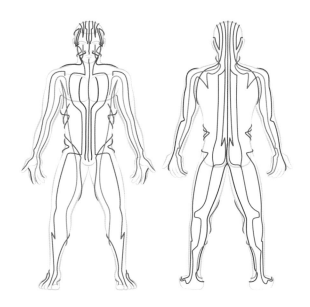

The Meridian System

A meridian (經絡) is a path or channel for Qi to flow. In TCM, we see the body as made up of twenty meridians, categorized into two groups. One group is the Twelve Major Meridians, which connect various physical functions, and the other is the Eight Extraordinary Meridians, which prepare the twelve organ meridians.

Imagine a map of the New York City subway system. Visualize the pathways as they weave in and out of each other. Now, imagine a similar, intricate system of channels inside of us. Add another layer on to this map that holds our mental, spiritual and emotional body. Altogether, these networks create one giant synergetic system. These pathways transport our Qi, Blood and nutrients just as the circulatory system transports our Blood.

"When energy flows freely through the meridians and the body's organs work in harmony, then there is no place for disease or illness."

—Nei Jing

The Twelve Major Meridians

There are twelve Major Meridians located on each side of the body, mirroring one another. Each of the meridians corresponds to an internal organ and connects to the Five Elements (page 24).

- **Liver Meridian:** regulates the female reproductive system, circulation of energy and maintains the flexibility of the ligaments and the tendons
- **Gallbladder Meridian:** regulates the removal and storage of toxins produced by the Liver
- **Pericardium Meridian:** regulates Qi that surrounds the Heart and protects the heart on a physical and emotional level
- **Heart Meridian:** regulates the circulation of Blood to all organs
- **Small Intestine Meridian:** supports digestion, water absorption, nutrient absorption and bowel functions
- **Spleen Meridian:** transforms and transports foods and fluids to all parts of the body
- **Stomach Meridian:** controls nutrient distribution and the extraction of nutrients from food
- **Triple Warmer Meridian:** regulates the metabolism of the body and promotes general wellness
- **Lung Meridian:** controls how energy is consumed and impacts the respiratory system

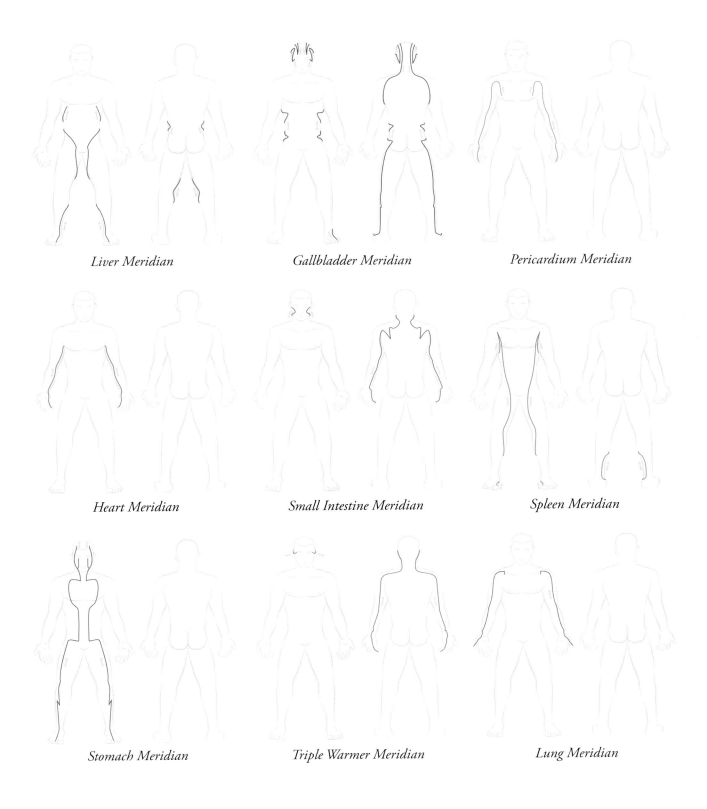

Liver Meridian

Gallbladder Meridian

Pericardium Meridian

Heart Meridian

Small Intestine Meridian

Spleen Meridian

Stomach Meridian

Triple Warmer Meridian

Lung Meridian

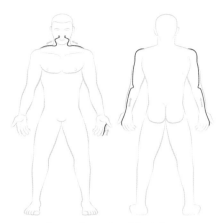

Large Intestine Meridian

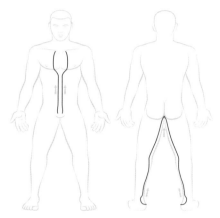

Kidney Meridian

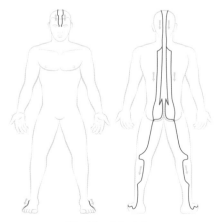

Bladder Meridian

• **Large Intestine Meridian:** regulates waste removal

• **Kidney Meridian:** regulates the reproductive system and testosterone levels, as well as produces bone marrow and Blood

• **Bladder Meridian:** regulates the removal of toxins from the body

The Eight Extraordinary Meridians

The Eight Extraordinary Meridians represent the energetic structuring at the body's deepest level. These are the meridians that are first to form before we are even born and they carry our inherited and ancestral energy. This energy is our genetic inheritance of deep energy, like a reservoir where the twelve main meridians can replenish themselves and also drain their excesses.

• **Du Mai:** The Governing Vessel

• **Ren Mai:** The Conception Vessel

• **Chong Mai:** The Penetrating Vessel

• **Dai Mai:** The Belt Vessel

• **Yang Chiao Mai:** The Yang Mobility Channel

• **Yin Chaio Mai:** The Yin Mobility Channel

• **Yang Wei Mai:** The Yang Regulating Channel

• **Yin Wei Mai:** The Yin Regulating Channel

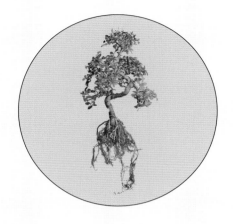

Chapter 3

Understanding Illness Through Traditional Chinese Medicine

Just as TCM offers a different lens on viewing your body, it offers an alternative perspective on viewing disease. Disease is not thought to be a completely random experience but more of an intentional one. Although that can seem much different than what you are used to thinking about disease, it can help reframe any helpless thoughts you may feel when experiencing symptoms or discomfort to put you in control of your health!

What Is Disease?

The notion of disease is thought of today mostly as something outside of us, something that is happening to us. It is presented as a separate entity of its own. We treat disease as a surprise and unwelcome guest that has entered our home and then try just about anything to kick out this perceived nuisance from our sacred space.

This notion must be looked at from a different angle and much closer, as we are missing the very message that the disease brings when it knocks at our door. In its simplest form, disease means "lack of ease," originating from old French. When we are at ease, we are in natural flow. As we have learned in TCM, free and natural flow equates to good health.

In Chinese medicine, when there is disharmony and imbalance of the functional entities, the major functions are unable to optimally perform, manifesting sickness. Disease is ultimately viewed as arising from an imbalance or a disruption of the flow of Qi and Yin-Yang rather than a purely physical phenomenon. When internal disharmony exists, disease manifests.

A pattern or syndrome is an integral part of understanding disease through a deeper perspective to find its root cause. A pattern helps us find the best course of treatment in TCM. Each disease has its own way of developing, in many stages, and is different for everyone. There is a Chinese proverb that translates as "different diseases, same treatment; same disease, different treatments."[1]

---

1   Zhai Xing et al., "Treating Different Diseases With the Same Method—A Traditional Chinese Medicine Concept Analyzed for Its Biological Basis," *Frontiers in Pharmacology* 11, no. 964 (2020): 26, 10.3389/fphar.2020.00946

In TCM, instead of focusing directly on the disease and attacking it as if it is a fight, we first focus on strengthening the organ systems, balancing the body and reestablishing harmony.

Many Symptoms, Same Root Cause

You will see in reading this book that a myriad of symptoms can stem from one root cause. For example, many headache types (page 86) and insomnia types (page 93) have the same root cause, even though they manifest in different ways depending on the person. Many different symptoms can be treated similarly, but the same symptom can be treated differently depending on the person, as the (root) cause can vary.

The Six Evils

Classified as the "Six Evils" (六淫), cold, fire, dryness, dampness, wind and summer heat are natural elements that are considered pathogenic when experienced to a certain degree. Originally observed thousands of years ago, we continue to refer to them in all aspects of TCM as they help us diagnose, treat and understand the patient.

These "evils" can originate both externally and internally through weather, seasons, choice of food, an individual's body constitution and lifestyle. Think about cold for example. Cold can be visible in ice cubes and snow, but there is also an invisible cold, one that can penetrate deeply into the body and manifest as a cold-to-the-touch body temperature, like chilling cold hands and/or feet.

If this still feels too abstract, keep reading. We are going to do a deep-dive into each element and start to learn why certain symptoms flare up for some individuals during specific weather patterns— arthritis when it's cold or rainy, fatigue on a humid day and a headache after being outside on a cold windy day.

- **Cold** (寒) damages our precious Yang energy and creates stagnation. It stops the flow. One thing to always remember in TCM is that our vital energy, Qi, and Blood (since they are inseparable) must always be flowing freely. Cold contracts, shrinks and stagnates Qi and Blood—limiting circulation. Symptoms like cold hands and feet are an example of internal cold. Because hands and feet are the farthest point that Blood and Qi need to travel, the symptoms are often felt there first. Chills, shivering, numbness, cramping and spasms can occur. Cold can attract other illnesses. Cold is associated with the Kidney system and the Water element.

- Just as heat rises, so does **Fire** (火), causing symptoms in the upper body, especially in the head, mouth and eyes. Fire is also referred to as heat, as heat is the manifestation of fire and fire is the nature of heat. Symptoms can happen at any time of the year and are not limited to warmer weather and are quite commonly experienced. The rising energy can disrupt the mind, and emotions like anger and irritability ensue. Fire also damages the body's fluids or Yin and fluid metabolism in the body through pushing out the fluid in the form of sweat. Symptoms experienced are irritability, red face, red eyes, sweating, extreme thirst and yellow phlegm. Fire can stagnate in local areas, causing sores, ulcers, redness, swelling, burning and painful sensations, especially in the mouth. Heat is associated with the Heart system and the Fire element.

- **Dryness** (燥) is related to the Lung system. The Lung and Large Intestine are responsible for moisture, the skin and the excretion of waste. The Lungs particularly are responsible for spreading our body fluids, also called Jin Ye. The word "Jin" means anything liquid or fluid. The word "Ye" means fluids of living organisms. Jin Ye equals organic fluid. Dryness damages Jin Ye, which is responsible for our tears, sweat, and organ lubrication for our brain and spinal cord fluid in the form of a "mist," which moistens skin and regulates the opening and closing of pores. Just like leaves can dry out and shrivel up, our body can experience dry cough, dry and cracked skin, dry hair, dry tongue, chapped lips, constipation, and sweaty hands and feet, along with the many uncomfortable symptoms of menopause like night sweats, low estrogen and vaginal dryness. The driest season is from the Autumnal Equinox to the Li Dong (beginning of winter), which is usually early November, and during Lung season. Dryness is associated with the Lung system and the Metal element.

- **Dampness** (濕) is heavy and sticky, a Yin substance that forms in the Spleen system and then is stored in different parts of the body, varying from organs to meridian systems. Dampness is the result of the digestive system's inability to assimilate food and transform and transport fluids. One of the key roles of the Spleen is to transform and transport fluid throughout the body. When that function is impaired, dampness is created. Dampness impairs Yang since it is considered a Yin substance. Certain foods, medications and body types are more prone to dampness and environments like humidity can be a contributor as well. Phlegm is seen as a condensed form of dampness forming over time. It creates a sticky, swamp-like environment. Once dampness accumulates, this buildup of sticky, heavy moisture brings stagnation to the rest of the body, which looks like fatigue, heaviness, edema, bloating, sluggishness, phlegm and excess weight. Dampness can be difficult to clear and that is why you will see it mentioned often as a cause of many symptoms. It is stagnant by nature, spreads easily and easily reoccurs. Imagine it like the gum on the bottom of your shoe in terms of how much of a nuisance it is to get that last bit of residue off! Dampness is associated with the Spleen system and the Earth element.

- **Wind** (風) is a Yang pathogen that we refer to as the leader of all evils. Although it is most experienced in the springtime, it is often the leading cause of disease. This is due to the nature of wind. Think about the times you've observed wind. Wind floats and disperses—it gusts and changes in severity rather quickly. In the body, the microcosm, it has the same characteristics. Headaches are the most common sign of wind, especially ones that seem to appear out of nowhere, just as a gust of wind easily comes and goes. Wind attacks are usually brought on quickly and could be at different places at different or the same times, usually manifesting in the upper parts of the body like the neck, shoulder, head, Lungs and back. Symptoms caused by wind are common colds, coughing, headaches, itchy skin, rashes, cramps, itchy eyes, joint pain, dizziness and involuntary shaking. Wind is associated with the Liver system and the Wood element.

- **Summer Heat** (暑) can occur during the "dog days of summer," as its property is hot and dispersing, a byproduct of consistent hot weather and/or the body not being able to adapt to a hot climate. This is usually the case in people with a weak constitution, as this type of heat can consume and deplete their Jin Ye (page 47). Symptoms that arise from being in extreme heat or prolonged heat are excess sweating, extreme thirst, lack of Shen, fatigue, heat stroke and dizziness. Extreme situations can cause fainting, loss of consciousness and cold limbs. It is best to avoid exposing yourself during the dog days of summer for too long. Summer heat is associated with the Heart system and the Fire element.

> *"The organs weep the tears the eyes refuse to shed."*
>
> —Sir William Osler

The Seven Emotions

Our emotions (七情), feelings, thoughts and physical health act as an interdependent cycle—and our emotions play perhaps the largest role. We seldom realize that our health affects our emotions or that with lifestyle and diet we can positively impact our emotions.

Emotions are considered to be the major internal cause of illness in TCM.

Emotional activity is a normal response to our external environment, yet, if any one emotion becomes overpowering, over time, it can cause serious damage to the internal organs. What causes the damage to the organ is a prolonged duration of emotion or an extreme emotion. Each one of us contains a different threshold for emotions, but once the organ systems are weakened, gateways open to imbalance, then symptoms and disease. This works as a cycle: The weaker a particular organ system is, the more susceptible one is to experience the associated emotions. And the more one experiences excess of a certain emotion, the weaker the system becomes.

Through understanding our emotions, we can work with this cycle to improve our entire well-being. Our emotional balance will improve and so will our physical symptoms. Remember, nothing is experienced out of coincidence.

Anger

A certain degree of anger can drive one to manifest positive, impactful change, as it can be the fuel to accomplish goals and draw out creativity. But just like all the emotions, excess leads to imbalance. In this case, an excess of anger, constantly being exposed to angry situations and suppressing anger can completely hinder one's health. Qi stagnation occurs.

When Qi is stagnated, so is Blood. The Liver is the organ system responsible for the smooth flow of these essential substances, as well as our emotions, so when this is hindered, the whole body is. An intense outbreak of anger can induce sudden headaches, dizziness, chest pain and other signs of Liver Qi moving upward in the body. Furthermore, anger can be rooted in wanting to obtain control. The Liver thrives on flexibility, as its element Wood is strong yet flexible to nature's ebbs and flows—it must bend to not break.

Joy

The standard meaning of joy is a great feeling because it is one of deep contentment. When joy consists of contentment, it promotes free and smooth-flowing Qi and a happy Heart. When joy becomes exaggerated, it turns to overexcitement to the point of agitation. Often, this can stem from desire and the craving for stimulation. Our modern lifestyles are quite stimulating on a day-to-day basis with technology, entertainment, alcohol, caffeine, nicotine and prescription drugs like Adderall and Ritalin. Constant stimulation does not let our Heart rest. We have glorified always being busy and have forgotten the importance of restorative rest. Overstimulation can lead to symptoms categorized as Heart fire and manifest as palpitations, insomnia, unclear thoughts, feelings of restlessness and agitation, talking incessantly and a red tip of the tongue. Qi disperses and the Shen becomes scattered. Over time, continued overstimulation can enlarge the Heart and weaken the pulse.

Worry and Overthinking

Worry is the associated emotion of the Spleen and the Stomach, the organs associated with the Earth element. The act of worry means dwelling too much on one thing in particular or concentrating on it too hard for too long, giving way to anxiety or unease. It is allowing one's mind to dwell on difficulty or troubles and negatives. This ends up creating more worry and anxiety, which is a vicious cycle and that's why it is hard for some to gain control.

If you've ever wondered why worrying is usually met with a stomachache, nausea or decreased appetite, you already know more about TCM than you thought. Just like we take in food and need to assimilate it, we do the same with our thoughts. Overthinking is essentially digesting the same thought over and over again. This repeated motion takes Qi to do. It uses quite a bit and, over time, it weakens the ability to digest food and emotions. This results in weak digestion and the accumulation of fluids and dampness, weighing you down physically, mentally and emotionally. Worry stagnates or knots Qi and depletes Blood. This leads to a weakened digestion, creating digestive issues, a lack of clear intention, brain fog, boredom and being unmotivated, and can be a vicious cycle, which creates anxiety.

Often, people who constantly worry have no appetite because their digestion has shut off. This then results in the body not being able to produce enough Blood because food is not metabolizing.

Grief

Grief is a feeling of deep sorrow, usually associated with the death of a loved one. Because there is no emotional meter on what grief really is—or the severity of it—what is felt by each person is completely individual. Grief is what happens internally, not what is reflected on the outside. For example, a relationship's end can tear someone's life apart, but another person can find it manageable.

Grief is the feeling associated with the Lung organ system. Our Lungs are responsible for taking oxygen into the body and breathing out air full of harmful carbon dioxide. They are responsible for taking in the new and letting go of the old along with their partner, the Large Intestine, which also expels waste. This partnership takes in the new (Lungs) and expels the old (Large Intestine). This system is all about letting go.

This partnership is most activated during fall, when nature itself lets go. Leaves on a tree fall and animals migrate or prepare for hibernation. TCM traditions teach us that humans are connected to and experience the same cycles as the natural world that surrounds us.

A normal and healthy expression of grief can be expressed through sobbing. This deep crying originates in the depths of the Lungs through deep breaths and expulsions of air with the sob.

If that urge to sob is suppressed, in many cases of severe and excess grief and sadness, disorders can arise in both the Lungs and Large Intestine. Symptoms like asthma, chronic coughing or shortness of breath can result from the Lungs withholding something that desperately needs expelling and constipation can result in the Large Intestine. In many cases of severe and excess grief and sadness, disorders can arise in both the Lungs and Large Intestine, as breathing issues and elimination issues go hand in hand. This applies to our emotions as well, as allowing new experiences and letting go of anything old or stagnant also go hand in hand.

Our will to be open and let in the new when one chapter ends and let go what no longer serves us is not only vital to our emotional stability but our physical bodies.

Fear and Fright

Fear is the emotion connected to the Kidney organ system and winter. Historically speaking, winter is the season connected to conservation and feelings of scarcity, a time people would be in survival mode to make sure they had enough of everything until spring. When we feel fear, our Qi descends, which correlates to that sinking feeling you've felt if you've ever been really scared. In extreme cases of fear, one can lose control of their Bladder (the Kidney's partner organ) and urinate themselves.

Above the Kidney system sits the adrenal glands, which release cortisol, the primary stress hormone that activates the sympathetic nervous system or our "fight or flight" response. This response helps us be alert to possible dangerous or life-threatening situations. The body physically reacts when it feels fear as well, curling inward to protect vital organs.

In our modern world, these hormones are more often activated when experiencing chronic stress or through traumatic situations. These instances create an energy leak and, since the Kidney system acts like the batteries of our entire operation, this leaves the body feeling depleted. Fear is normal and adaptive, but if it becomes chronic, then an imbalance begins and one may feel emotions like a lack of willpower, insecurity, aloofness and isolation.

Furthermore, winter is the most Yin of the seasons, as it is the coldest and darkest. Yin is slow-moving, the pace is intentionally allowing complete reflection and introspection, which can be quite scary to surrender to. In our society, we are constantly on the go and we seldom take time to slow down because of apprehension to what we may find when we do.

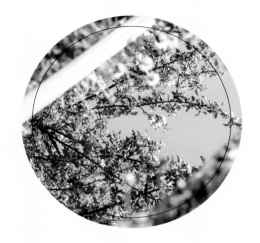

Chapter 4

Healing Methods

The following methods are the most practiced healing modalities in TCM. Each one uses the foundational aspects we've covered so far, like Qi (page 20), Yin and Yang (page 16), meridians (page 42) and the organ systems (page 24) as a guide for healing. The great news is that you can practice methods like acupressure (page 52) and gua sha (page 53) at home and find certified acupuncturists or Chinese medicine doctors in your area to perform acupuncture and prescribe herbal medicine.

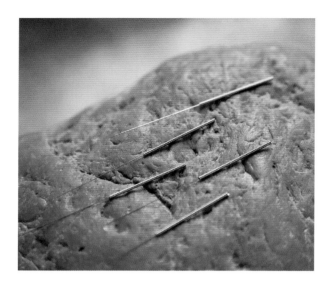

For example, point Large Intestine 4 合谷 He Gu (LI4), translates to "Union Valley." "He" means close together and "Gu" means between two mountains or valleys. The space between the index finger and thumb forms a valley and that is where you find point LI4. Union Valley indicates a place where more than one valley connects, so this point tells us that lots of Qi and Blood in the Large Intestine are abundant, collected and stored in the valley. Therefore, this point is used to treat so many discomforts, ailments and symptoms, ranging from chronic and non-chronic pain, headaches, facial problems, wrinkles and can even be used for numbing the body for surgery. I always call this point Grand Central Station—it can connect to anywhere.

Acupuncture

Acupuncture (針灸) is directing the flow of Qi, or energy, through the body with very thin needles. This concept originated in China, first recorded in documents dating back thousands of years ago. Before needles, sharpened stones and bones were used.

The first document that unequivocally described an organized system of diagnosis and treatment recognized as acupuncture is *The Yellow Emperor's Classic of Internal Medicine*.

Acupuncture points are like mini landmarks that support the body's functioning in specific ways. Each point contains a specific name and meaning. The acupressure points are measured by "cun," or the Chinese inch, and it is proportionate to one's own body. The ancient sages used intentional and descriptive names for each point to instill the wisdom to the practitioner of their specific purpose and healing capability.

Acupressure

If you've ever worn a motion sickness wristband or pinched the skin between your thumb and index finger for tension relief, you've performed acupressure (指壓) on yourself and didn't even realize it.

Acupressure is an ancient form of massage. It is the practice of applying manual pressure to the same energy meridians and acupoints as those targeted with acupuncture to move our vital Qi into a specified meridian channel. By moving the Qi and opening the flow of it, it can get where it needs to for healing, pain relief and nourishment. Acupressure is a wonderful alternative or addition to acupuncture and is a noninvasive practice you can learn and do at home.

In Part 2 (page 56), I will show you many acupressure points to help the associated conditions covered in this book.

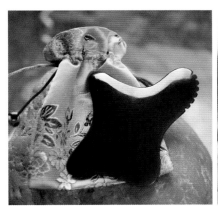
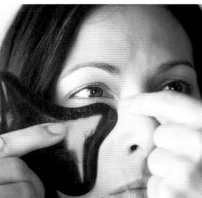
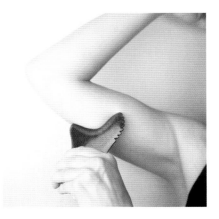

Gua Sha

Gua sha (刮痧), pronounced "gwah-shah," originates from the Chinese word for scraping. It can also be referred to as spooning or coining, as a traditional soup spoon can be used. Classically, a gua sha tool is made from jade, horn or bian stone. The treatment for gua sha is done by using the tool to apply pressure on the skin using a stroking motion. Depending on the pressure used and how the individual reacts, temporary bruising can result. The small bruises caused by gua sha are sometimes known as microtrauma, which creates a healing action in the body to help break up scar tissue. Commonly, people experience pain where there is scar tissue due to lack of fresh Blood. Qi is unable to reach the desired area as the scar tissue creates too many small, blocked pathways.

Gua sha has been used to dissolve tension, aches and pains; prevent chronic disease; invigorate proper organ function; increase immunity; boost circulation; improve metabolism; and move Blood and Qi through meridian channels. Pain in the body is experienced when Qi is blocked or stagnant, so this ancient method aims to move energy around the body. It also helps to break down scar tissue and connective tissue, improving movement in the muscles and joints.

More recently, gua sha has gained notoriety in the skin care world for its use on the face as a natural alternative to Botox. When made with the right material, like jade, it offers many benefits to facial appearance. Gua sha can invigorate Blood and Qi to the face, dissolve swelling and move out stagnated fluids for a youthful appearance. Because everything has intention in TCM, when made with authentic material like jade, the qualities and minerals also benefit the skin.

Chinese Herbal Formulas

Chinese herbal medicine (中藥方劑) has been utilized for thousands of years. It incorporates ingredients from all parts of plants—the leaf, stem, flower and root. Each part of the plant can often have different effects on the body and, for that reason, each part is used intentionally and with care.

Herbs are similar to acupuncture in terms of the tremendous effect they can provide to the body. Nature supplies us with what we need: If nature creates a symptom, nature creates a remedy.

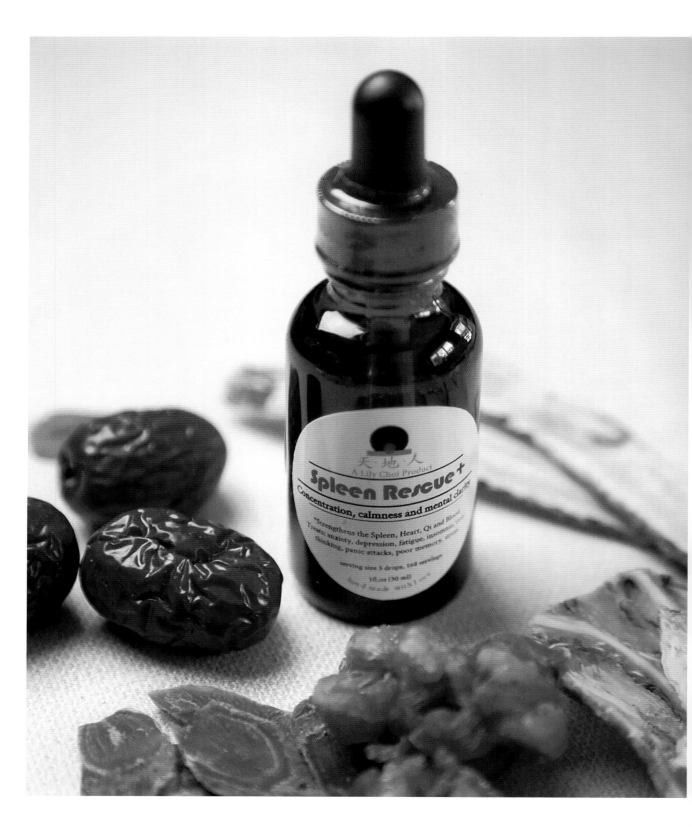

Herbal decoction is a method of extraction done by boiling herbal or plant material to dissolve the chemicals, which may include stems, roots, bark and rhizomes. This can be an arduous process, but it is one of the most potent ways to consume herbs and that is why I started creating my very own herbal tinctures.

I wanted my patients to take herbs without having to make time-consuming decoctions or figuring out how to source the best-quality herbs, so I began making tinctures for them to use with ease. Being able to help my patients and my community with these formulas allows me to continue my father's legacy in a profound way. If you're interested in browsing the tinctures I make, you can do so on my website (lilychoinaturalhealing.com).

In Chapter 6 (page 113), I put the spotlight on several of my favorite herbs that help an array of ailments. Most herbs are taken in combination with other herbs. In addition to taking herbs together in a formula, there are some herbs that work wonderfully on their own and I highlight some of my favorite single-use herbs as well.

Meditation and Qigong

All of the branches of TCM work together to provide total support to all the bodies: mental, physical and emotional. Meditative and Qi-building exercises are just as integral as the physical methods of healing.

Meditation (冥想) offers balance to the body both in the moment when you're meditating and over time when you practice regularly. Immediate benefits can include a lowered heart rate and increased relaxation. Long-term benefits can include enhanced immune function, increased ability to focus and an overall sense of well-being.

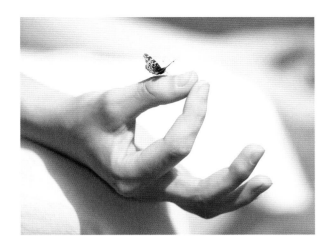

Qigong (氣功) is a combination of two concepts: "Qi," which is the vital life force energy of the body, and "gong," which is the skill of working the Qi. Together, Qigong means cultivating energy. Any practice that can cultivate Qi is not one to be overlooked.

Qigong can be described as a mind-body-spirit practice that improves one's mental and physical health by integrating posture, movement, breathing techniques, self-massage, sound and focused intent. There are likely thousands of Qigong styles, schools, traditions, forms and lineages, each with practical applications and different theories. Chinese archaeologists and historians have found references to Qigong-like techniques from at least 5,000 years ago!

The benefits of Qigong include lowered stress and anxiety, increased focus and improved balance and flexibility. It may even reduce your risk of certain chronic diseases. You can look up a style of Qigong that resonates with you online or locally source a practitioner that teaches Qigong in your area.

"You should sit in meditation for 20 minutes every day—unless you're too busy. Then you should sit for an hour."

—Zen proverb

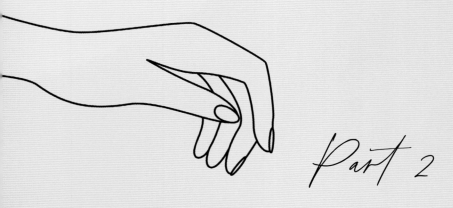

Part 2

TREATING ILLNESSES, CONDITIONS AND HEALTH ISSUES

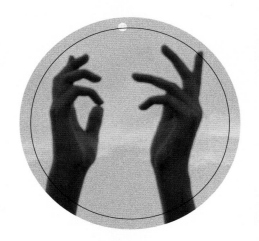

Chapter 5

The Root Cause of Common Conditions and Ways to Heal

In this next chapter, I've detailed the most effective methods for healing the symptoms I see most commonly in my practice. We'll go through emotional ailments, physical conditions and chronic diseases. I'll help you to understand them through TCM and offer methods of healing each one. When on your healing journey, be patient, but, ultimately, be consistent! Remember how long it took you to get where you are and, although the body's natural state is to be healthy, it will take persistence and patience to reach homeostasis.

Acid Reflux

Gastroesophageal reflux disease, or GERD, is more commonly known as acid reflux. It is categorized as a digestive disorder that affects the ring-shaped muscle called the lower esophageal sphincter found between the esophagus and the stomach. When the liquid in the stomach regurgitates, or refluxes into the esophagus, a burning pain ensues. The burning pain in the chest usually occurs after eating and worsens when lying down. Symptoms of acid reflux, in addition to varying severities of heartburn, may include coughing, asthma, chronic bronchitis, nausea and a sore throat. Often, those suffering don't see much improvement in their overall condition of GERD with prescribed or over-the-counter antacids.

What Causes This?

In TCM, we know that GERD is the body letting us know of a deeper, underlying imbalance. The most common imbalance resulting in GERD is a disharmony between the Liver and the Stomach organ systems. From the Five-Element Framework (page 24), we know that the Liver supports the Spleen and the Stomach systems. If the Liver Qi (energy) becomes stagnated either through emotions or toxins, it lashes out on the Stomach.

Harmonious digestion is a result of our Liver Qi flowing upward and outward while the Stomach Qi flows downward. Together they create balance, allowing for a smooth and pain-free digestive process. If this harmony is consistently interfered with, acid reflux and many of its accompanying symptoms can result.

Harmonious Flow

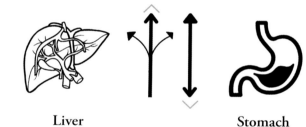

Liver   Stomach

Disharmonious Flow

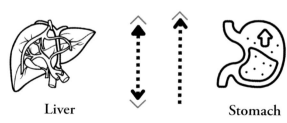

Liver   Stomach

How Is This Harmony Most Interfered with?

• **Emotions like stress and excessive worrying.** Stress affects the Liver and interrupts the smooth flow of Liver Qi, not allowing synchronistic flow with the Stomach and creating that unpleasant acid reflux in the esophagus. Think about it like digesting the same thought repeatedly. This weakens Stomach function and can lead to GERD.

• **Toxin accumulation from lifestyle, environment and diet.** The Liver system oversees detoxing the body. Habits like overworking, poor diet, staying up late and stimulant abuse make the Liver unable to detox properly, stagnating the flow of Liver Qi and resulting in disharmony between the Liver and digestion.

How to Heal

Foods and Herbs

• Consume ginger. The phenolic compounds can help relieve gastrointestinal irritation and lessen gastric contractions. Ginger is used to reduce the likelihood of acid flowing from your Stomach back into your esophagus. Drink my Ginger Power Tea (page 125) twice daily before 6 p.m. until symptoms ease up, then use it daily for maintenance.

• Focus on your digestion. Eat a warming breakfast daily (page 113) and focus on a diet of whole foods with consistent mealtimes. Avoid eating late at night, alcohol, tobacco, refined sugars and processed foods.

Lifestyle

• Receiving consistent acupuncture treatments with a licensed practitioner can effectively inhibit the intraesophageal acid and bile reflux in GERD patients to alleviate symptoms.

• Practice flexibility. Our Liver system correlates to the element Wood (page 28). Wood is strong, yet it ebbs and flows in accordance with the wind, so it doesn't break. Nature demonstrates to us that wood requires flexibility in order to survive. Often, as humans, we want to have control over situations in our life. I ask you to work toward finding the balance between control and going with the flow and you will find much improvement in your symptoms.

Acupressure

• **Pericardium 6** 內關 "Inner Pass" is located between the tendons of the inner wrist, three fingers from the inner crease of the wrist. This point has many amazing uses, helping acid reflux, heartburn and nausea. When you stimulate the point along the meridian, it helps send signals of energy to promote digestion and calm the body.

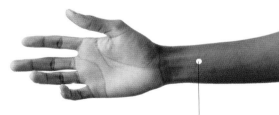

Pericardium(PC6)

Acne (and Other Skin Conditions)

Acne is the most common skin condition and can be stressful to deal with not only physically but emotionally as well. It is an inflammatory skin condition usually caused by an excess of oil, bacteria and dead skin clogging the pores. There are several types of acne and it can manifest on many parts of the body.

Although we are only going to cover the topic of acne, many skin conditions like eczema, psoriasis and dry skin can be helped similarly to how we treat acne.

Our skin is our largest organ and we can use it as a barometer to get an idea of what is going on inside the body. The skin is a mirror that reflects the internal environment.

What Causes This?

In TCM, acne is most related to Stomach and Spleen deficiency. This weakness in the digestive system creates a condition we refer to as damp heat. In the Six Evils (page 46) section, we spoke about dampness and heat separately, but they can form together to create damp heat.

The equation that leads to acne can be a sum of the following: consumption of spicy, greasy, sugary and oily foods; stress that affects hormone levels; medications; lifestyle habits like sweating without wearing breathable clothing; personal hygiene; and face masks can also contribute to bacteria formation.

This pathogen travels through the meridians and acne can form on the face (especially on the chin) and on the back. In this case, the ability of the Lungs to open and close the pores becomes impaired. This hinders the natural detoxication of toxic dampness and heat, so acne forms because the waste isn't expelled.

No matter why or where your exact type of acne manifests, the following treatment can help harmonize the root imbalance.

A Closer Look at Skin Conditions

Although every organ influences the skin, the skin is the tissue associated with the Lung and the Large Intestine systems and is referred to as the "third Lung." Just as we discussed the Lungs being our first defense from the outside world (page 36), the skin does just that, creating a boundary between our inner and outer worlds.

The main focus with any skin condition is to make sure the Spleen and the Lung systems are strong. If you remember from the Five-Element Framework (page 24), the Spleen system is the generator of the Lung; if the Spleen is weakened, the Lung function will be too.

How to Heal

Foods and Herbs

• Avoid greasy, oily, fried and barbequed foods. Dairy can also play a role in acne formation, so it is best to avoid it and see how that elimination affects the skin.

• Invigorate Spleen function by eating breakfast daily, reducing the amount you worry and eating simple to digest foods so that dampness can be relieved. Refer to the recipes in Chapter 6 (page 113) to support you.

• Self-Heal (page 137) is an herb that is great for acne because it relieves heat, which affects the Spleen and the Lung systems contributing to the condition.

Acupressure

• **Stomach 36** 足三里 Zusanli "Leg Three Miles" is an essential point for Spleen deficiency and helps relieve dampness greatly while supporting the Lungs. This point is located below the kneecap, roughly 3 inches (7.5 cm) below and 1 inch (2.5 cm) away from the center of the body. To massage this point, place two fingers on the points. Apply gentle but firm pressure to the points with both fingers, it most likely will feel tender. Rub daily for several minutes on each leg. Drink warm water afterward.

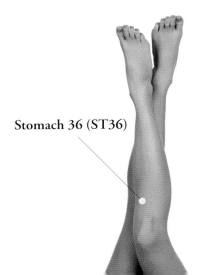

Stomach 36 (ST36)

• **Large Intestine** 4 合谷 He Gu "Union Valley" is located in the mound between the thumb and index finger. Rub each hand for several minutes every day. *Do not use this point if you are pregnant, as it can induce labor.*

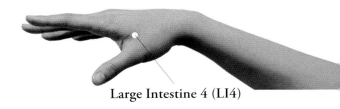

Large Intestine 4 (LI4)

Lifestyle

• Be mindful of bacteria reinfection. If you are suffering from acne, make sure to always use clean towels, pillowcases, clothing—whatever touches your face. A great tip to prevent reinfection is to iron your pillowcase for 10 minutes before bed.

• Focus on going to bed early, relieving stress naturally, managing emotions and reducing your toxic load, which all help to reduce heat.

Allergies

Allergies are a great example of the "We Are Mini Universes" concept (page 13). Allergies are triggered by either external (environmental) or internal (one's own body) forces or a combination of both. This shows us how well our mini-universe (our body) is in harmony with the larger universe and how well we can adjust to our ever-changing environment.

What Causes This?

There are three primary channel pairings with the most influence on the complexity of allergies:

- **Lung and Large Intestine:** Metal element, Fall
- **Spleen and Stomach:** Earth element, Late Summer
- **Liver and Gallbladder:** Wood element, Spring

The Lungs provide our immunity and are our first line of defense, protecting us from illness and helping fight it off. When the Lung system is harmonious, it protects us from colds and allergies. The Large Intestine is the partner to the Lung and the Stomach is the partner to the Spleen, and both of their meridians run through the nose and sinuses. A stuffy nose or congestion in the head signals you to look to those organs. When the Spleen can't regulate digestion and dampness forms, symptoms of runny nose arise. And the Liver channel connects to the eyes, so any eye discomforts have to be treated through the Liver.

The Spleen and the Stomach generate the Lung. Late summer is the time when the Spleen and the Stomach are highlighted by nature. If they are imbalanced or weak, they will not be able to support any problems the Lung may experience. If they are strong, they can help the Lung overcome weakness during the fall.

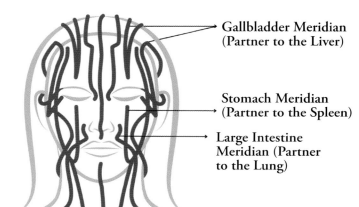

Gallbladder Meridian (Partner to the Liver)

Stomach Meridian (Partner to the Spleen)

Large Intestine Meridian (Partner to the Lung)

How Internal vs. External Factors Influence Allergies

- **External factors:** Many of the Six Evils (page 46) contribute to allergies, mostly wind, dryness and cold. Each of these natural environmental elements relate to a specific organ and a time of year. For example, if you feel as though your allergies flare up in the spring, there is a correlation to the element of Wind and the Liver system, as that is the system most energized in spring. For allergies in the fall season, it is more about dryness and Lung function. These elements can invade and affect the body if it is unable to adjust to its changing environment.

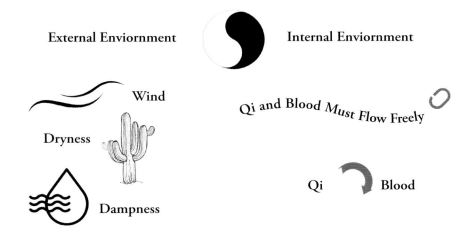

External Enviornment

Internal Enviornment

Wind

Dryness

Dampness

Qi and Blood Must Flow Freely

Qi   Blood

- **Internal factors:** External factors do not affect everyone the same, as some people are more resilient to them. The body is unable to digest whatever the allergy is, meaning it is lacking sufficient Qi to perform its job or flow. Because the Kidneys carry our inherited essence, as well as act as our body's battery pack, those suffering from allergies usually have a weaker constitution or a bit of Kidney deficiency, meaning the Kidney system could stand to be strengthened! Check page 38 to learn more about the Kidney system.

How to Heal

Foods and Herbs

- Eat a warm breakfast daily (page 113) and replace any cold or iced drinks with warm tea or warm water to boost digestive function. Also, avoid greasy, processed and packaged foods that are harder to digest and will clog your digestion. A well-functioning Spleen system will help your allergies!

- Spirulina is blue-green algae that has been researched to help inflammation-driven reactions, like seasonal allergies, by blocking histamines. One placebo-controlled study found that spirulina successfully decreased symptoms of allergic rhinitis, including nasal discharge, sneezing, nasal congestion and itching.[1]

- Local bee pollen contains enzymes, nectar, flower pollen, wax and honey. It contains anti-inflammatory, antimicrobial and antifungal properties. With consistent use, bee pollen can help build resistance to the kind of pollen in your environment that is affecting you. Make sure the pollen is local.

---

1   Cingi Cemal et al., "The effects of spirulina on allergic rhinitis," *European Archives of Oto-Rhino-Laryngology* 256, no. 10 (2008): 1219-1223, 10.1007/s00405-008-0642-8

Allergies (continued)

- According to research, taking probiotics can help reduce symptoms of allergic rhinitis.[2] Probiotics help balance gut flora to provide us with immune support and to combat any potential inflammation that is present with allergies. Probiotic-rich foods include sauerkraut, kimchi, fermented or pickled vegetables, miso and natto, which is a fermented soybean product popular in Asia.

- Herbs like goji berries (page 133), astragalus (page 130) and schisandra (page 136) are also found to very much benefit intestinal bacteria.

Acupressure

- **Large Intestine 4** 合谷 He Gu "Union Valley" is located in the mound between the thumb and index finger. This is a miraculous point that can treat all head and face issues. Use it for headaches, red or itchy eyes, fevers, heat in the face, sinus troubles and for an immune boost. It moves Qi and Blood stagnation to stop pain. *Don't use this point if you are pregnant.*

---

2 Zajac Alexander et al., "A systematic review and meta-analysis of probiotics for the treatment of allergic rhinitis," *International Forum of Allergy & Rhinology* 5, no. 6 (2015): 524-523, 10.1002/alr.21492

- **Large Intestine 20** Ying Xiang 迎香 "Welcome Fragrance" has long been used to treat disharmonies of the nose, such as rhinitis, sinusitis, allergies, loss of smell, nasal discharge, sinus issues, nasal polyps, facial paralysis, headaches and common colds. Located on either side of the nostril, it can also help those who are suffering from loss of smell. Rub this area with the base of your thumbs, where you can pair up with another impactful point, **Lung 10** 魚際 "Fish Border." This point is located midway between the bottom of the thumb and the wrist, where the palm meets the thumb (right where the skin color changes).

Lifestyle

- Good air quality is important to maintain in general for less stress on the Liver and the Lungs. A good-quality, high-efficiency particulate air filter will remove pollen, dust and pet dander particles from the ambient air. This works best if you also make sure to keep windows and doors closed when you suspect pollen is heavy in the air outside.

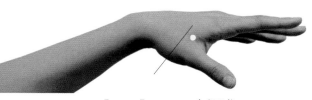

Large Intestine 4 (LI4)

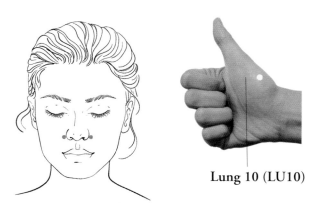

Large Intestine 20 (LI20)

Lung 10 (LU10)

Anxiety

Anxiety is defined as a feeling of fear, dread and uneasiness about everyday situations. Immediately, this definition lets us know it should not be common, as it is far from the natural universal harmony we are looking to connect to.

Although the phrase "anxiety disorder" did not originally exist in TCM terminology, its manifestations are very similar to conditions treated for thousands of years. Anxiety is approached not so much as a brain dysfunction, but more as an inner organ dysfunction that affects our thoughts.

What Causes This?

Anxiety affects the Zang organs—Heart, Lung, Spleen, Liver and Kidneys—and each organ system has associated feelings of anxiety. If any of the below manifestations resonate with you, circle back to the Five-Element Framework section (page 24) where the organ systems—and ways to strengthen them—are outlined in full. Because anxiety is rooted in fear and fear-based thinking, we do want to pay close attention to the Kidney system, which is associated with fear (more on that on page 39).

- **Heart Manifestations:** lack of enthusiasm or vitality, mental restlessness, depression, insomnia, despair. The Heart is always treated in cases of anxiety because it stores our Shen (page 20), which is loosely translated to our spirit and mind.
- **Lung Manifestations:** grief, sadness, detachment
- **Spleen Manifestations:** worrying, dwelling or focusing too much on a particular topic; excessive mental work

- **Liver Manifestations:** anger, stress, resentment, frustration, irritability, bitterness and "flying off the handle"
- **Kidney Manifestations:** fear, insecurity, aloofness, isolation, weakness, not much willpower

How to Heal

Food and Herbs

- Refined sugars can cause wild fluctuations in blood sugar and insulin levels, which can significantly affect one's mood and mental health. Refined sugars also deplete B vitamins from the body, which can affect the nervous system.
- Especially avoid stimulants like alcohol, tobacco or e-cigarettes.
- Excessive amounts of caffeine can create heat in the Liver, which rises upward in anger and anxiety. As an adrenal stimulant, caffeine can ultimately lead to adrenal exhaustion and depression. Substituting refined sugar and caffeine with low-glycemic foods and beverages can result in reduced anxiety.

Anxiety (continued)

• Nourish your Yin energy to cool the body down internally with wild yams, black beans, organic non-GMO tofu, black wood ear mushrooms, black dates, snow mushroom, mulberries, lotus root and pears.

Acupressure

• **Heart 7** 神門 "Spirit Gate" is located on the wrist crease at the pinky side and is the point for emotional issues, especially excessive anxiety and worry. The Spirit Gate point offers us the door to access our spirit, mind and emotion. Press strongly until you take a deep breath and repeat on the other wrist. Repeat as needed.

• **Yin Tang** 印堂 "Hall of Impression" is one of the "extraordinary points," which means it stands on its own and is not part of any particular meridian. Yin Tang is located in between the eyebrows, at the point associated with the "third eye." Touch the spot between your eyebrows with your index finger or thumb. Take slow, deep breaths and apply gentle, firm pressure in a circular motion for 5 to 10 minutes.

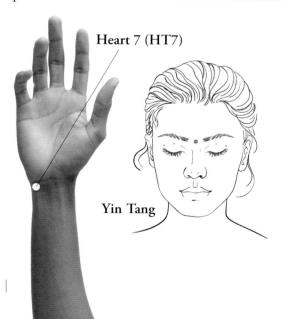

Heart 7 (HT7)

Yin Tang

Lifestyle

• Meditation, therapeutic practices and Qigong can improve your health from the inside out, offering a different perspective on events and occurrences in your life. They are not to be overlooked or dismissed. These practices can help you quiet the mind, understand yourself on a deeper level and experience more compassion for yourself and others, as well as forgiveness and an opportunity to address any emotions or feelings that have been suppressed.

• Consciously make the effort to disengage from screens and virtual realities, especially 2 to 3 hours before bed. Spend the time to be where you are, to connect to yourself with the practice of gratitude. Avoiding blue light (the kind of light emitted from screens) before bed is essential for a good night's sleep, as more than any other color, blue light blocks the hormone melatonin that makes you sleepy. A good night's sleep is imperative for cognitive function, stress, emotions, digestion and detoxification.

• A practice that has been around for centuries called "grounding," also referred to as earthing, is the simple act of making contact with the earth, specifically with your bare feet. Making contact with the macro earth can very much help the micro earth inside of you: the Spleen and the Stomach. Mentally, grounding is said to aid in the reduction of stress, anxiety and depression. It can also help to improve focus and concentration, increase feelings of calm and improve your mood and overall well-being through the absorption of negative ions. Negative ions are molecules floating in the air or atmosphere that have been charged with electricity. Since we are energetic beings and our Qi rules us, this can serve as a recharge.

Arthritis

Arthritis is a degenerative condition that affects the joints. In Western medicine, it is categorized as an inflammatory condition of one or more joints, which can worsen with age. The two main types of arthritis—osteoarthritis and rheumatoid arthritis—damage joints in different ways.

Osteoarthritis is the most common type of arthritis and occurs when the joint's cartilage wears down over time and can also be brought on prematurely by a joint injury or infection. Cartilage is the cushion at the end of the bones that allows for smooth joint motion, but, when damaged, it results in bone grinding on bone, which causes pain and affects range of motion.

Rheumatoid arthritis is an autoimmune disease where the body destroys the joint capsule, a tough membrane that encloses all the joint parts. This lining becomes inflamed and swollen. The disease can eventually destroy cartilage and bone within the joint.

What Causes This?

In TCM, arthritis is referred to as bi syndrome. Pathogenic wind, cold, dampness and/or heat creates meridian obstruction and sluggish Blood and Qi circulation. This creates pain, stiffness and/or swelling. Certain people are more susceptible to bi syndrome than others. In older people and those with a weak constitution, invading pathogens can usually penetrate deeper. Each person will experience the pathogens at a varying degree, creating a complex array of symptoms that can be completely different for everyone.

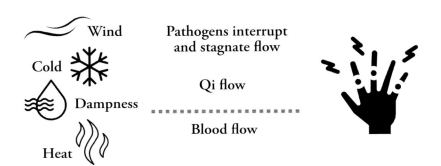

Arthritus (continued)

How to Heal

Foods and Herbs

• Have Ginger Power Tea (page 125) daily to reduce inflammation and help expel cold, wind and dampness. Ginger invigorates Spleen function for stronger muscle tone.

• Foods high in zinc like oysters, crab, lobster, red meat, chicken, turkey, beans and nuts can help, as studies show significantly lower zinc levels in people with rheumatoid arthritis compared to those without.[1] The lowest levels are associated with more severe disease. Researchers say zinc may help improve rheumatoid arthritis symptoms by supporting the immune system and cartilage.[2]

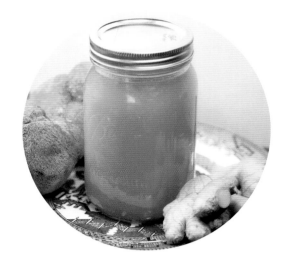

• Cherries, especially tart ones, have been recorded to show relief in the pain and stiffness one can experience with osteoarthritis. Cherry juice or a handful of cherries daily will do the trick. Berries like blueberries, raspberries, strawberries, cranberries and blackberries contain anthocyanins, which reduce inflammation, and ascorbic acid (a form of vitamin C), which is quite helpful.

• Eat a diet rich in natural collagen and collagen-boosting foods (not powders) like Bone Broths (page 121), black wood ear mushroom, chicken feet soup (or add chicken feet to your bone broth), schisandra (page 136), wild yam, vitamin C, garlic, pumpkin seeds and berries.

• Avoid inflammatory foods, iced drinks and over-consuming raw and cold foods, which slow down the flow of Qi and Blood.

• Drink Light as a Feather Tea (page 129) to drain dampness during the warmer weather months, as resolving dampness will improve arthritis conditions.

• Use San Qi (page 135) to treat inflammation and arthritis, as well as benefit from the herb's neuroprotective effects to help any associated nerve pain.

1   Mierzecki Artur et al., "A pilot study on zinc levels in patients with rheumatoid arthritis," *Biological Trace Element Research* 143, no. 2 (2011): 854-862, 10.1007/s12011-010-8952-2
2   Khanna Shweta, "Disease-Modifying Antirheumatic Diets: The New Treatment Modalities for Rheumatoid Arthritis," *European Medical Journal* 5, no. 1 (2018): 93-99, 10.33590/emjrheumatol/10312960

- Burdock root contains fatty oils along with sterols and tannins to make this herb very anti-inflammatory. It also helps to drain dampness. You can eat burdock root in stir-fries, supplement with it or make a decoction. To make a decoction, chop 2 tablespoons (15 g) of fresh burdock root or use 2 teaspoons (5 g) of the dried root as an alternative. Add the root to the boiling water and allow it to simmer for 10 minutes, then turn off the heat. Strain and drink while still warm. Three to four cups (720 to 960 ml) a day is ideal.

- Avoid spicy foods, deep-fried foods, barbecued foods and greasy foods because they reduce the body fluids that moisten our skin, joints and organs.

- Additionally, for rheumatoid arthritis, also avoid gluten and nightshade vegetables until your symptoms subside. Nightshades are a family of plants that includes tomatoes, eggplant, potatoes and peppers, which can cause inflammation and achy muscles and joints. They also contain solanine, a calcium inhibitor.

Lifestyle

- Consistent and moderate exercise practice is crucial for those dealing with arthritis, as it increases strength and flexibility, reduces joint pain and helps combat fatigue. Low-impact aerobic activity, strength training and balance exercises should be cycled for complete care.

- Reduce or change positions of the affected joints to reduce the pain in those areas and make sure to wear supportive shoes if you have arthritis in the lower joints.

- Massage the affected joint area with herbal oil to help activate circulation around the area. Ginger extract applied topically also helps.

- Research has shown that acupuncture has benefits for rheumatoid arthritis, osteoarthritis and chronic pain because of its ability to open the flow of Qi and Blood. Furthermore, acupuncture can manage pain by boosting the number of endorphins, or natural painkillers, your body makes.[3, 4]

- Avoid icing the painful area. In TCM, we don't put ice on an injury or on pain because ice restricts the flow of Blood. Healing occurs with fresh Blood flow to the area. Ice impedes the natural healing process, ultimately prolonging recovery and increasing the likelihood of the injury recurring. After icing, cold can easily become trapped in the weakened area, leading to aches and pains after the injury is gone. This can prolong arthritis and create more pains later on.

3 Zhang YuJuan and Chenchen Wang, "Acupuncture and Chronic Musculoskeletal Pain," *Current Rheumatology Reports* 22, no. 11 (2020): 80, 10.1007/s11926-020-00954-z

4 Patil Shilpadevi et al., "The Role of Acupuncture in Pain Management," *Current Pain and Headache Reports* 20, no. 4 (2016): 22, 10.1007/s11916-016-0552-1ache reports vol. 20,4 (2016): 22. doi:10.1007/s11916-016-0552-1

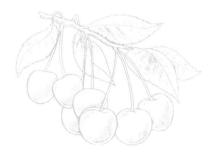

Candida and Parasites

Parasitic disease has been a problem for humans since the beginning of time. Did you know that almost every culture has their own remedies and preventative measures to manage parasites? Whether it be garlic, wormwood, cloves, pumpkin seeds, ginger, herbs or administering colonics, there were always natural measures being taken to prevent illness caused by parasitic activity.

Why do we have to worry about parasitic disease? Because most parasitic infections do not create a serious health threat, they are largely ignored by modern medicine. In TCM and more and more in all arenas of functional and integrative medicine, parasites are said to be the cause of many common ailments, anywhere from fatigue and irritable bowel syndrome to skin issues. If left untreated, they can develop into larger issues. Do note that the point of being aware of parasites is to manage them and make sure they do not become overpopulated, as they will never be completely eradicated.

What Causes This?

Parasites are more active during the new and full moons, which was mentioned in *The Criterion of Evidence and Governance (Standard of Diagnosis)* in the 1600's Ming dynasty. It says that the "most efficient times to kill parasites are during the new moon and full moon, other times their heads and body are down and hiding, so is not as effective."

Around the full moon, parasites increase movement in their host (yup, that would be us humans and our furry pets). Our circadian rhythm is affected by the moon. We produce more serotonin and less melatonin, which creates an ideal breeding ground for these smart and stealthy bugs, as they hide within the deep tissues of our organs and come out during these periods.

Toxin-wise, another problem with parasites is that when they overpopulate, they take on heavy metals from the system. There are frequent correlations between those with a higher number of parasites carrying a larger heavy metal burden. Heavy metals bind to parts of your cells that prevent your organs from doing their job. The average person most likely has more heavy metals in their body than they realize. For example, pesticides and herbicides that are sprayed on our food (which are hard to completely avoid even on a strict organic diet) are a common source of heavy metals.

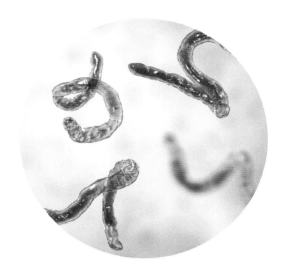

A Closer Look at Candida

Candida overgrowth is a more commonly recognized fungal infection. Candida infections can occur in people of all ages and in different parts of the body. Candida albicans is the species of candida fungus or yeast that most often naturally appears in the body. It can manifest in the mouth and is known as thrush or on the genitals and is known as a yeast infection. When it's kept at normal levels in the body, it aids in digestion and in the absorption of nutrients from food. When the levels of this fungus grow out of control, however, digestive problems of all sorts can be triggered and the standard practices of eating, digestion and elimination are ruffled.

TCM views candida overgrowth as a result of Spleen deficiency creating the pathogen dampness (page 47). When dampness collects in the pelvic region, it creates phlegm and leads to congestion and heaviness. This is what can lead to vaginal yeast infections or prostate problems.

How to Heal

Foods and Herbs

• Focus on strengthening the Spleen system through your diet and resolving dampness (page 47) first rather than on detoxing. When you strengthen the Spleen system, you improve intestinal mobility to move out parasites and any unwelcomed guests.

• Ginger and its constituents play a vital role in the prevention of microbial growth or act as antimicrobial agents. In addition to using ginger in your cooking, in Chapter 6 (page 113), I will discuss my favorite way to have ginger.

• For a pilot study published in the *Journal of Medicinal Food* in 2007, sixty children with intestinal parasites received immediate doses of either an elixir containing a mixture of papaya seeds and honey or honey alone. After seven days, a significantly greater number of those given the papaya seed–based elixir had their stools cleared of parasites.[1] To eat papaya seeds, just scoop 1 teaspoon of raw seeds, grind them and consume them in your food.

---

1 Okeniyi John A O et al., "Effectiveness of dried Carica papaya seeds against human intestinal parasitosis: a pilot study," *Journal of Medicinal Food* 10, no. 1 (2007): 194-196, 10.1089/jmf.2005.065

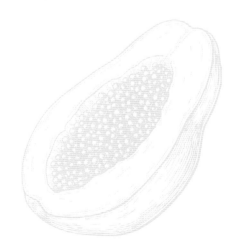

Candida and Parasites (continued)

- Key spices and foods to incorporate in your diet are pumpkin seeds, garlic, oregano, oregano oil, cloves, wormwood, raw onions, radicchio, raw garlic, thyme, rosemary, cayenne pepper, coconut oil, coconuts and cinnamon.

- Probiotics are live bacteria and yeasts that are good for you, especially for your digestive system. It is essential to rebuild and maintain healthy and beneficial gut bacteria. You can do so by eating probiotic-rich foods like miso, sauerkraut, kimchi and natto. You can supplement with a high-quality probiotic daily. This is a crucial step for people who have taken many antibiotics throughout their life.

- Although cloves are most used as a culinary spice, they are great and effective for parasite management as some of the active compounds in clove buds are powerfully anthelmintic (antiparasitic).

- Increasing your consumption of carrots, sweet potatoes, squash and other foods high in beta-carotene, a precursor for vitamin A, is said to increase your resistance to penetration by parasites.

- Spirulina (preferably from Hawaii) is an algae that draws out heavy metals from the brain, central nervous system and Liver, and it can protect the body from parasites and cleanse them from the system.

- While being cognizant of parasites, stay away from sugar, coffee, refined sugar, alcohol and refined grains. This is what they love to feed on. Notice your cravings around the full and new moons, you may find that you crave those foods then. Furthermore, avoid raw meats, fish and shellfish.

Lifestyle

- Take care of your pets and practice good pet hygiene, as our furry friends carry parasites and can transmit them to us.

- Infrared saunas emit infrared light on your skin for assistance in deep healing, as the rays penetrate the body, thus helping Blood flow, detoxification assistance and the removal of toxins.

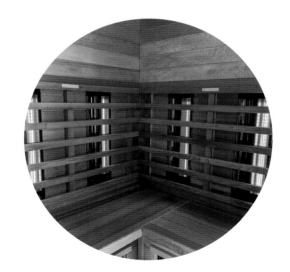

Cold Hands and Feet

Cold hands and feet can be an uncomfortable and even puzzling condition—especially if you experience this sensation when it's not even cold outside! The poor circulation of Blood can cause cold hands and feet, but there are different reasons for this weak circulation. Through understanding the main causes, you can help eradicate this symptom and boost your body's energy to finally feel warmth all over. According to Western medicine, iron deficiency, anemia and poor circulation are the main causes of cold hands and feet, which is a direct correspondence with TCM.

What Causes This?

In its simplest form, cold hands and feet can be thought of like a break in your body's internal energy circuit. Various energetic imbalances (like deficiencies and stagnation) can create a break in the circuit of proper circulation. This means poor Blood circulation in the limbs is a result of energy depletion. In this situation, the body reduces Blood supply to less important areas such as the digestive tract, hands and feet in order to safeguard supply to critical organs such as the brain and Heart.

Circulation is connected to Blood. As discussed on page 23, Blood is a greater concept in TCM than it is in Western medicine, as it is considered a Yin substance that nourishes and moistens all the organs, muscles and tissues. When the extremities are cold, it signifies that both Qi and Blood are unable to reach the areas farthest from our Heart. This can signify that Blood is lacking or not in free flow. For cold hands and feet, Qi and Blood flow must be invigorated.

When the Liver becomes distressed over a period of time, it can cause Blood to become stagnant, since the Liver stores Blood and is responsible for keeping everything moving freely and easily in our bodies.

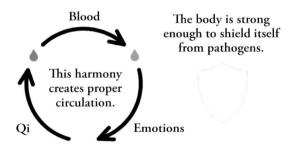

Blood

The body is strong enough to shield itself from pathogens.

This harmony creates proper circulation.

Qi

Emotions

Common Symptoms from Different Imbalances

• **Yang Deficiency:** feelings of extreme cold under whatever circumstances, tendency to have loose stool, back and knee soreness, often feeling tired or fatigued and women could have white discharge

• **Qi and Blood Deficiency:** pale face; easily tired; anemic; menstrual issues like painful, scanty or short periods

• **Liver Qi Stagnation:** cold hands and feet but the body doesn't feel cold; feeling constantly stressed, angry and/or frustrated

How to Heal

Food and Herbs

• Eat a diet full of strengthening and hot foods. This includes chicken, beef, beef liver, lamb, scallions, dark leafy greens, ginger, sesame seeds and longan fruit.

• Avoid all cold drinks, ice water and raw foods. Eat warming foods (read more on this on page 35).

• Booster and Builder Tea (page 126) can improve Blood circulation, expel dampness and promote healthy Qi.

• Eat warming spices like cinnamon, turmeric, black pepper and cayenne pepper.

• If you identify with the above description of Liver Qi stagnation, add plenty of green vegetables to your diet and cook them with my simple sauté method (page 117).

Lifestyle

• Moxibustion is a specific method of heating specific acupuncture points on the body by burning an herb called "moxa" close to the skin at specific acupoints. This therapy is so valued that it is said that when all else fails to heal, you can rely on moxibustion. This herb can be purchased in stick form online or done by your practitioner. Please keep in mind the moxa is very hot and the stick and ash can burn you if it touches your skin. Procced with caution when using it.

• Sunbathe the back and spine daily (weather-permitting) for 5 to 20 minutes.

• Soaking your feet daily promotes Blood circulation and enhances the flow of Qi. Foot soaks are a common Asian practice with many health benefits. Soak your feet daily for 15 to 20 minutes. You can also add cut-up and smashed ginger to the bath to increase the warming energy available.

• If you identify with the description of Liver Qi stagnation, manage emotions and workload, reduce stress and don't snack or eat too close to bedtime. Meditate daily, go to bed before 11 p.m. and practice consistent, moderate exercise.

Constipation

Constipation is a condition in which you may experience infrequent bowel movements; stools that are hard, dry or lumpy; stools that are difficult or painful to pass; or a feeling that not all stool has passed.

There are several patterns of imbalance that can lead to recurring or prolonged constipation. Usually, there is more than one pattern present at the same time for those dealing with constipation that is not a result of situational causes. Those include travel, pregnancy, diet change, certain medications and ignoring the urge to go to the bathroom. Certain conditions like thyroid disease, Parkinson's disease or stroke can lead to constipation as well.

What Causes This?

In modern medicine, if we have a problem like constipation, we may take a laxative or any number of medicines to target movement in our colon. In Chinese medicine, we take it one step deeper and say that colon imbalances often originate with the Lung. The main reason being that the Large Intestine is the partner of the Lung (read more about this partnership on page 36).

Yin is our fluids and our moisture. When there's a deficiency, it leads to insufficient fluid to lubricate the intestine and heat results from the lack of moisture, therefore drying the intestine and stool. Blood is a Yin fluid essential for proper bowel movements, so those with Blood deficiency (page 23) can experience constipation.

Patterns of Constipation and Their Related Symptoms

- **Excess Type** is the most common type of constipation resulting from an excessive Liver energy, which generates heat or stagnation. Liver heat dries up body fluids, which leads to dry and hard stools, dry mouth, frequent thirst with aversion to heat, bad breath, bloating, reddish complexion or a yellow coating on the tongue.

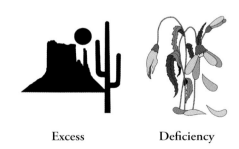

Excess   Deficiency

Constipation (continued)

- **Deficiency Type** is the result of lack of Yin fluids and/or Blood in the body, which leads to dry stools that are difficult to expel, paleness in the face, dizziness, hot flashes, night sweats, forgetfulness and the tongue may lack coating. Additionally, it can include headaches around the menstrual cycle or painful periods.

How to Heal

Food and Herbs

- Make sure your diet is full of fiber. Fiber-rich foods include avocados, berries, pears, Brussels sprouts, artichokes, lentils and edamame.
- Incorporate hydrating foods like Congee (page 114) and Bone Broths (page 121) into your daily diet.
- Hydrate with warm water to open the flow of Blood and Qi. Avoid cold drinks.
- Foods like rice, millet, seaweed, black beans and beets help to increase Yin fluids.
- Avoid dry foods like crackers, toast and chips, which contribute to heat and further remove moisture from the intestines.
- Astragalus (page 130) is a super-herb adaptogen, which has the ability to boost Qi and tonify Yang. You can boil dried strips of astragalus in tea or in your next pot of bone broth or use it in extract form. It's best for the deficient type.

- Black sesame seeds are a beloved ingredient and superfood in TCM and I refer to them often in this book. They contain a high fiber content and unsaturated fatty acid content. The oil found in the seeds can lubricate your intestines, while the fiber in the seeds helps with smooth bowel movements. Take 1 to 2 tablespoons (9 to 18 g) per day, grind them with a mortar and pestle or a coffee grinder and use the powder to top your Congee (page 114), soup or blended drink.
- Aloe vera juice, dandelion greens and the Self-Heal herb (page 137) can help for temporary relief. It's best for the excessive type.
- Drink Rice Water (page 118). The nutrients in rice water help relieve constipation and provide the Spleen and the Stomach with quick, usable energy.

Supplements

- Magnesium helps to increase the amount of water in the intestines, which can help with bowel movements, especially a magnesium supplement that includes magnesium oxide, citrate and succinate.

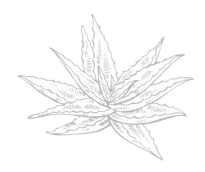

Lifestyle

• Exercise invigorates an otherwise sluggish digestive system and regular movement will tone up the muscles and reflexes for those who are weak. It can also help to burn off Liver excess and boost fluid metabolism.

• The Large Intestine is associated with "letting go." If you suffer from constipation, on some level there is an emotional tie to being unable to get rid of thoughts, feelings or situations that are no longer serving you. In this case, you want to take action to remove physical clutter from your space, donate old clothing and assess if you're holding on to anything deeper.

• Emotions like anxiety, stress or worry interfere with the body's natural ability to eliminate. If you experience these emotions along with constipation, don't rush off the toilet. Instead, take your time, don't take your phone with you to the toilet and take deep breaths to allow the whole body to relax.

• Enemas are injections of fluids used to cleanse or stimulate the emptying of your bowel by way of your rectum and they can be administered at home to provide temporary relief. Please check with your practitioner to see if it is suitable for you. If you do practice this method, make sure to add many probiotic foods into your diet for the days following the enema. They include sauerkraut, kimchi, miso, spirulina and wild sea moss. These probiotic-rich foods are beneficial even if you don't perform an enema. This is best suited for the excessive type but can be used for the deficient type, just not frequently.

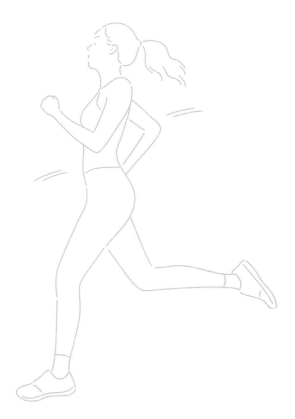

Digestive Issues

Most people experience digestive issues of some variety at some point in their life. Some conditions are more chronic, while others may flare up from time to time with seemingly no rhyme or reason. Digestive issues are a large umbrella term to cover many of the most common symptoms such as bloating, poor digestion, IBS symptoms, gas and abdominal pain.

What Causes This?

• If we have **Spleen Yang deficiency** or low Spleen energy, our digestive fire is weak, impairing our immunity, metabolism and ability to digest. This can often manifest as diarrhea, bloating, loose stool, undigested food in stool, feeling cold often and having trouble metabolizing food, thoughts and emotions.

• **Liver stagnation** is the other main cause of digestive issues. The moving function of the Liver regulates proper Qi flow in the entire body and influences the way the other organ networks function, particularly the Spleen system. According to the Five-Element Framework (page 24), the Liver supports Spleen function. If the Wood element (the element associated with the Liver, page 28) becomes imbalanced, either by being overcharged or stagnated, it will unleash on the Earth element (associated with the Spleen, page 33) and impair its functioning. Therefore, many digestive issues affecting the Spleen and the Stomach generate through Liver dysfunction.

Liver stagnation often manifests as irritable bowel syndrome symptoms, being easily agitated, bloated, constantly sighing, rib pain, fullness and tightness in abdomen, anger, vomiting, nausea, diarrhea, poor digestion, premenstrual syndrome, amenorrhea, insomnia, hair loss, mouth sores, chronic gastritis, chronic cholecystitis and chronic enteritis.

Liver System

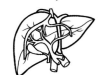

Spleen System

Controlling

How to Heal

Food and Herbs

• It has been said to "eat breakfast like a king, lunch like a prince and dinner like a pauper." Our Qi moves through the body cyclically, also known as our circadian rhythm or body clock, so different organs are more energized at different points of the day. The Stomach and the Spleen function optimally in the morning between 7 and 11 a.m., needing hot and fresh fuel to power the immune system, build Blood, supply cognitive function, warm the body and have proper energy.

• Avoid cold and raw foods. Food is transformed by our digestive fire and this fire dims when we constantly ingest cold drinks and raw foods. Choose warming and Spleen-enhancing foods like ginger, sweet potatoes, pumpkin, wild yam, rice and soups.

• Eat seasonal foods. We want to live in harmony with our natural environment as much as possible. Ideally, we want to eat what is local, seasonal and fresh. When we focus on the food in season, we offer a greater healing support to our bodies.

• Focus on proper chewing. Digestion begins in the mouth. Breaking down larger particles of food into smaller particles reduces stress on the esophagus, helps the Stomach metabolize food and increases digestive enzymes. It sends messages to the digestive system to trigger hydrochloric acid production, helping food move through the digestive tract. What's the magic number? About twenty chews per bite. It may be hard at first, but keep practicing and activate your muscles. This also helps strengthen the facial muscles!

• The Spleen is nourished by mild sweet flavor and damaged by extreme sweetness from processed foods and refined sugars. Constant sweet cravings are a common sign of a Spleen imbalance. When you focus on natural sweet-essence foods like carrots, sweet potatoes, parsnips and squash, you will notice less cravings and feel more satiated.

• To heal digestive imbalances, focus on the 清淡, which means "Light and Simple Diet." Read more about this principle on page 113.

Lifestyle

• Avoid multitasking. When the eyes are engaged in other activities like reading, watching television or looking at your phone, it weakens the Liver system, as the Liver governs the eyes. The Spleen enjoys mindfulness as opposed to multitasking.

• Emotions play a starring role in our digestion! Any one of the Seven Emotions (page 48) can hinder our ability to digest food and cause unpleasant symptoms of nausea and diarrhea and trigger more chronic conditions.

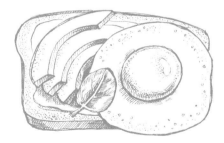

Fatty Liver

Nonalcoholic fatty liver disease (NAFLD) is the accumulation of liver fat in people who drink little or no alcohol. Standard medicine states that the cause of NAFLD is unknown, but risk factors include obesity, gastric bypass surgery, high cholesterol and type 2 diabetes. Most people have no symptoms; therefore, the disease remains severely under the radar.

Fatty liver disease affects between 90 to 100 million people in the United States and 17 percent of children. Considering the standard American diet, it is no wonder the rates have reached this height: The largest contributor to NAFLD is the consumption of processed foods and sugars, not fat. When sugar is consumed, lipogenesis occurs, which is the metabolic formation of fat, the body's normal response to sugar.

NAFLD creates inflammation that leads to Liver disorders like steatohepatitis and cirrhosis of the Liver. Heart attack risks increase because high triglycerides develop and the good cholesterol (high-density lipoprotein) reduces. Diabetes and obesity are also related to NAFLD due to the inflammation created by this disease. Practices like Blood tests and ultrasounds can detect NAFLD.

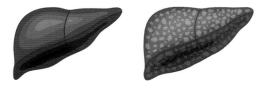

Deposits of fat can cause liver enlargement.

What Causes This?

According to TCM, NAFLD is created from a pattern of Spleen deficiency because of dampness formation and Liver Qi stagnation.

A weak digestive system results from the pathogen dampness (page 47), as sugars, sodas, and refined and processed foods are all damp-forming foods creating a slow, heavy and turbid digestive environment. Dampness, a phlegm-like substance, disrupts the healthy flow of Qi and Blood and creates stagnation, disharmony and eventually disease in the Liver.

How to Heal

Foods and Herbs

• Cut out processed foods, which include sugar, soda and anything containing high-fructose corn syrup and refined sugars. Avoid processed foods or foods in packages!

• Reduce starches. Refined white flour and even foods labeled as "whole grain" or "wheat" are a problem, as they can be loaded with sugars. Instead, try organic sweet potatoes, yams, potatoes and white rice in small quantities, all of which are healing. White rice is sometimes labeled as controversial in Western diets, but, in TCM and many other cultures, white rice is very healing for the Spleen and expels dampness when consumed in moderate amounts. For example, Congee (page 114) can invigorate digestive function.

• Eat fats like grass-fed beef, beef liver and wild salmon.

• Goji berries (page 133) have been a superfood in TCM for thousands of years and are now being studied for their miraculous benefits, specifically dealing with the Liver. Research has said that they can even promote Liver regeneration. Research on animal models indicates goji berries can help with managing liver health and preventing the progression of alcohol-induced fatty liver disease.

• Eat good fats like olive oil and avocados. Consume dark leafy greens like artichokes, dandelion greens, kale, collard greens, mustard greens, Swiss chard, broccoli, Brussels sprouts and cabbage.

• The Liver loves sour foods. This is the taste correlated to the organ, so include plenty of lemons, limes, apple cider vinegar and fermented foods like sauerkraut and kimchi, which can promote Liver detoxification. Daikon radishes, onions, garlic, milk thistle and turmeric also work well.

• Ginger Power Tea (page 125) increases Yang energy, powering the body to remove toxins, promote circulation and increase immunity and metabolism. This directly supports Liver function.

• NAC (N-Acetylcysteine) is a potent amino acid that increases glutathione levels for Liver detoxification. Bone Broth (page 121) is an excellent source of NAC too and can further help Liver and Spleen healing.

• Magnesium and B vitamins also provide tremendous support to the Liver.

Acupressure

• **Liver 3** 太 "Supreme Rushing" is a powerful point, as it enables Qi to move more freely around the body, stimulates the Liver and unblocks stagnant Qi. You can easily find this point in the web at the top of the groove between the first and second toes. Use the thumb to press and massage this point on both feet every day or you can use your opposite heel to stimulate the point while you sit. Practice this daily.

Liver 3 (LV3)

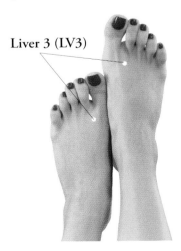

Fatty Liver (continued)

Lifestyle

• Get moving! We all know the importance of regular exercise. Working up a sweat helps the body detox naturally and release toxins stored in the Liver and helps to combat inflammation. Although you cannot exercise yourself out of a bad diet, consistent and daily moderate movement improves insulin resistance and reduces fatty liver.

• Manage your stress levels. Stress especially impacts the Liver, as stress results in elevated levels of the stress hormone cortisol and pro-inflammatory bio-markers, which could be involved in the development of NAFLD.

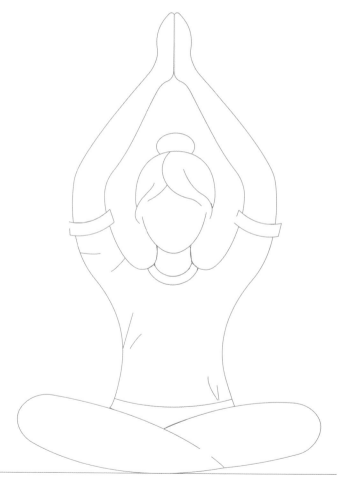

Hair Loss and Gray Hair

Although hair loss or graying of hair is typically associated with advancing age, an increasing number of people of all ages are experiencing this more so than ever. There are endless supplements, topical treatments and vitamins marketed to improving this condition. TCM offers wonderful support for restoring your crowning glory. Hair is used as a marker because it is a direct manifestation of our internal environment, one closely tied to the health of our Blood.

"髮為血之餘" translates to "The condition of the hair is a reflection of the condition of the Blood."

—*The Yellow Emperor's Classic of Internal Medicine*

What Causes This?

Hair will be healthy if there is sufficient Blood in the body because our Blood contains the nutrients required to nourish our hair. Blood is governed by the Spleen and Liver, so when those organ systems are smoothly functioning, hair will grow to be lustrous and strong. The Kidney system plays a crucial role in any side effect of aging as it governs the process. It also influences the growth of all body cells, including hair.

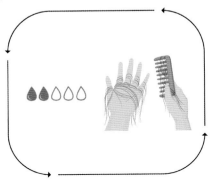

The Most Significant Root Causes of Hair Loss

- **Kidney Jing Deficiency:** Our Kidneys store our energy—think of them like the batteries of our body. When the batteries are overused and not properly recharged, the battery energy drains quicker, resulting in premature gray hair. This occurs from lifestyle habits like severe stress, overwork or overexertion, and living a "burning the candle at both ends" lifestyle.

- **Liver Blood Deficiency:** This occurs to those who are imbalanced from being overly busy, easily angered and overstressed. These lifestyle habits and ones like going to bed late affect the Liver Blood. It's a pattern that can also be common in females, especially those postpartum or ones who are vegan or vegetarians. For postpartum women, an ample amount of Blood and Qi are used during the birthing process, which can affect hair growth. For vegetarians, they may not be getting some of the essential amino acids and B vitamins only found in animal products. Any which way, the Liver Blood is unable to make it to the crown of the head and, therefore, unable to nourish the scalp.

- **Oily Scalp:** Another common cause of hair imbalances, oily scalp usually results from an unhealthy diet, such as the consumption of excessive sweet, oily, fatty, greasy or fried foods that result in dampness (page 47). Genetic reasons, improper hygiene and overprocessed chemical products, as well as stress, worry and nervousness can lead to endocrine disorders creating an overly oily or even a dry scalp. A healthy diet is a must to prevent the condition from getting worse and reversing the dampness and toxins in the body.

How to Heal (Tips to Help All Patterns of Hair Loss)

Foods and Herbs

- Black sesame seeds have been added to modern hair care products, but they have been used for quite some time as a standard TCM practice to combat grays. In TCM, black sesame seeds are known for their antiaging effects, as they nourish the Kidney system. Their black color signifies the Kidney's affinity toward them, as foods that are black in color benefit the Kidney system. The antioxidants found in black sesame seeds can help combat damaging the cells, which causes gray hair, hair loss and wrinkles.[1] Black sesame seeds contain nutrients that are nourishing for the scalp and boost melanocyte activity to produce melanin, the pigment in your hair that determines hair color. Take about 1 tablespoon (9 g) of the seeds daily. Buy them whole, not already ground, and grind them yourself prior to consumption to make sure you are getting the most out of these powerful little seeds.

- He Shou Wu (何首烏) is a popular remedy that is derived from the fo-ti (Polygonum multiflorum) plant and loosely translates to "the black-haired Mr. He" in Chinese. This herb supports and strengthens not only the Kidney organ system but also the Liver organ system. This name comes from Mr. He, a 58-year-old man from Hebei province of China. After seeking advice on what to take for his fertility, he started taking this herb daily. After a few months, he was able to father children, became more youthful and it was said he lived well over 100 years old with black hair. He Shou Wu has a restorative property essential to the Kidney system and to the Blood, with studies confirming that it can stimulate hair growth, as well as restore the color and sheen of the hair.[2] This herb is the main ingredient in my tincture called Follicle Power available on my website (lilychoinaturalhealing.com).

- Blood-building foods nourish the Liver and the Kidney system. Dark green leafy vegetables, chlorophyll-rich foods like spirulina and seaweed, beets, dark berries and red meat (especially organ meat) all have this capability and contain iron and vitamin B-12. Iron and vitamin B-12 are essential for healthy hair and are found in dark green leafy vegetables, iron-rich meats, nuts, beans and seeds. Vitamin B-12 is found in eggs, poultry and meat. If you are a vegetarian, it may be helpful to get vitamin B-12 in supplement form.

2 Bounda Guy-Armel and Feng Y U, "Review of clinical studies of Polygonum multiflorum Thunb. and its isolated bioactive compounds," *Pharmacognosy Research* 7, no. 3 (2015): 225-236, 10.4103/0974-8490.157957

1 Fereidoon Shahidi, Chandrika M. Liyana-Pathirana, Dana S. Wall, "Antioxidant activity of white and black sesame seeds and their hull fractions," *Food Chemistry* 99, no. 3 (2006): 478-483, 10.1016/j.foodchem.2005.08.009

- Omega-3 fatty acids are particularly important for a healthy scalp and can be found in mackerel, wild salmon, oysters, sardines, anchovies, walnuts, soybeans, and chia and flax seeds. You will see here that many of these foods are seafood. In TCM, salty foods and foods grown in salt water are the flavor most beneficial to the Kidney system.

- Mulberries (page 134) are beneficial for Yin energy and Blood tonification. They are often used to help prevent hair loss and early gray hair because of their ability to tonify (strengthen) Blood. The fruit can be eaten or taken in supplement form.

Acupressure

- Massage your head for 5 to 15 minutes, four to five times weekly. Use the tip of your finger pad. This stimulates and energizes the meridians in the head leading to increased Blood flow. You can also stimulate the scalp by brushing with a wooden comb, which is practiced in TCM to stimulate Blood flow to the crown of the head.

- For hair loss, you will want to stimulate two essential points simultaneously. **Kidney 3** 太谿 "Great Stream" and **Gallbladder 39** 懸鐘 "Suspended Bell." Kidney 3 is located on the inner side of the ankle, in the depression between the tip of the bony bump at the attachment of the Achilles tendon. Gallbladder 39 is located about four finger widths above the external ankle bone on the anterior border of the fibula. These points strengthen the meridians essential to our hair and get the energy where it is needed, up to the scalp. Rub points GB39 and KI3 at the same time with a good amount of pressure. Do it once or twice daily for 1 to 2 minutes each time.

Lifestyle

- Use Rice Water (page 118) topically. Studies have found that inositol, an ingredient found in rice water, is able to penetrate damaged hair and repair it from the inside out. It even protects hair from future damage. It is easiest to put it in a squeeze bottle if you want to use it on your hair. Use it after shampoo and conditioning. Rice water can detangle, smooth, shine and strengthen hair.

- Avoid going to bed with wet hair. This is an age-old practice in Asian cultures and many European cultures as well. When I moved to the United States, I was shocked to see how many people go out with wet hair and then I learned how people go to sleep with wet hair as well. In TCM, night is considered Yin time, meaning Yang energy is at its lowest. Energy is low at bedtime and, when Yang is low, the ability to resist pain is low as well. When you wash your hair before bed, water stays in the scalp, creating Qi (energy) stagnation and the stasis of Blood flow, blocking the meridian.

- Going to bed early, before 11 p.m., allows the Liver and the Gallbladder to sufficiently detox, promoting better Qi and Blood flow and helping emotional conditions like stress, which plays a large role in hair loss and the premature graying of hair.

- Take care of your eyes! The overuse of our eyes affects the Liver, damaging the Liver Blood, which can create hair loss. If you are on your cellphone and computer all day, make sure to make goji berries (page 133) a part of your daily diet. An eye exercise to perform every morning is to warm your hands and cover your eyes. Rotate the eyeballs clockwise thirty-six times and then repeat counterclockwise thirty-six times. This will help your eyes and hair!

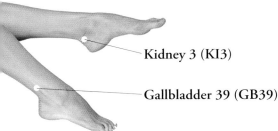

Kidney 3 (KI3)

Gallbladder 39 (GB39)

Headaches and Migraines

Let's first get to know our head. The head is connected to the internal organs through the meridians and branching channels. The head connects directly to the external organs through the eyes, ears, nose and mouth. When internal and external factors hinder the flow of Qi and Blood in the meridians, headaches can manifest. TCM classifies the head as "the convergence of Yang" because all the body's primordial energy, or Yang Qi, connects toward the head and the Yang meridians of the arms and the legs also pass through the head (page 42).

What Causes This?

There are more than 700 combinations of factors that lead to headaches, which have been recognized as eight patterns. Factors such as food, stress, dehydration and weather can lead to headaches. Hormones are also a culprit, especially for migraines in women. You can also suffer from more than one headache pattern.

Keep in mind for those with recurring headaches, it takes time to alchemize the root problem. Keep practicing the techniques I've outlined and they will help. These patterns can be used for migraines as well.

Before we get into the specifics of healing the eight patterns, here are some overall headache tips to start with: Avoid going to bed with wet hair (read more about this on page 85) and supplement with magnesium, especially if you suffer from migraines.

The Eight Headache Patterns and How to Heal Each

1: Liver Yang Rising

- **Headache Pattern:** distending and dizzy sensations, throbbing, pulsating, pounding and bursting feelings; aggravated by anger or emotional stress and has a tendency to affect the side of the head, temples, eyebrows or behind the eyes.

- **Accompanying Symptoms:** irritability, easily angered, dry stool, vertigo, red eyes, nausea, vomiting and throat dryness. There may also be tinnitus (ear ringing), discomfort in the low chest and difficulty falling asleep.

- **Emotions:** Calm the Liver. This is done through a variety of techniques, the largest being emotional balance. Stress, anger and frustration play a large role in this type of headache. Think about quite literally "What and who is my headache?" Do you find yourself getting this type of headache in a specific scenario or when you have a certain obligation? There is always an emotional connection. Alter your boundaries to match the needs of your body, as your body is signaling that there is a discord between your mind and your Heart. Write out your feelings daily, as you may not be expressing them fully.

- **Lifestyle:** Meditate daily and go to sleep before 11 p.m. Unplug from technology well before bed to allow your mind to peel back the layers from the day. What do you feel? Where do you feel? Express your feelings by writing them out so they don't stay stored inside of you.

- **Acupressure:** Use your index and middle fingers to press and release on point **Gallbladder 8** 率谷 "Valley Lead" on both sides. GB8 is located directly above the highest point of the ear, ½ inch (1.3 cm) from the top of the outside of the ear. Press and release quite vigorously on and around the point for 3 to 5 minutes as needed. Point **Liver 3** (find the diagram on page 81) is also very beneficial for this type of headache.

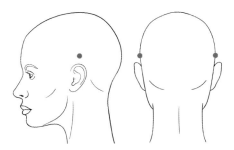

Gallbladder 8 (GB8)

2: Qi Deficiency

- **Headache Pattern:** lingering and dull pain in the whole head that is triggered or aggravated by fatigue or physical activities. It may not happen often. Those who are overworked or exhausted tend to develop this type of headache, along with those with weakened Spleen and Stomach function. Other organ systems can be weak as well, but low digestion is most common.

- **Accompanying Symptoms:** sallow complexion, shallow voice, fatigue, no appetite, sensitivity to cold, loose bowels, sweating easily, palpitations, puffy tongue.

HOW TO HEAL

- **Lifestyle:** Boost your vital Qi through building back up your body's strength with proper rest, moderate exercise, meditation, and consistent and healthy meals. See if there are activities and responsibilities that you can take off your plate to free up more of your energy.

- **Foods:** Avoid eating sour, cold, raw, oily and greasy foods. Focus on easily digestible and warm foods (page 113) with consistent mealtimes and don't skip breakfast. Have Ginger Power Tea (page 125) daily to boost the body's Qi.

- **Herbs:** Use astragalus (page 130) as a tincture, as tea or add it to your favorite soup or broth. This herb is one of the most Qi-tonifying things we can ingest. Do note that if you suffer from autoimmune conditions, it is best to talk to your doctor prior to use.

- **Acupressure: Stomach 36** 足三里 Zusanli "Leg Three Miles" is an essential point for Qi deficiency and helps relieve dampness. This point is located below the kneecap, roughly 3 inches (7.5 cm) below and 1 inch (2.5 cm) away from the center of the body. To massage this point, place two fingers on the points. Apply gentle but firm pressure to the points with both fingers. It most likely will feel tender. Rub daily for several minutes on each leg. Drink warm water afterward to flush out any stagnation.

3: Excess Dampness

- **Headache Pattern:** heavy feeling in the head and body, low appetite, aggravated by greasy or heavy foods, nausea, dizziness, vertigo, sinus congestion and pressure, brain fog, lethargy, abdominal distention, greasy yellow or white tongue coating. May be recurring.

- **Accompanying Symptoms:** joint pain or discomfort, skin issues, may suffer from cysts, fibroids, endometriosis, weak muscle tone, mucus.

HOW TO HEAL

- **Lifestyle:** Emotions and feelings that can result in dampness include persistent negative self-talk, as well as chronic worry, which affect the transporting and transforming function of the Spleen and lead to an imbalance in fluid metabolism.

- **Foods:** Implement proper eating habits and avoid skipping meals, especially breakfast. Refer to the warming foods and simple and bland diet (page 113). Avoid cold drinks, iced water or smoothies, as they dim the digestive fire. Avoid dairy and sugars as you heal from this condition as they greatly contribute to dampness (page 47).

- **Acupressure: Spleen 9** 陰陵泉 "Yin Mound Spring" is one of the most impactful points for relieving dampness. To locate this point, place a finger at the inside of your ankle bone and trace it all the way up the tibia bone until you meet resistance, right below the inside of the knee. In that little depression is Spleen 9 and it is typically a bit tender when pressure is applied. Rub this point on both legs every day. Stimulate for 30 seconds and then rest, repeating three to four times on both sides. Begin doing this gently and work your way up. Make sure to drink plenty of warm water afterward.

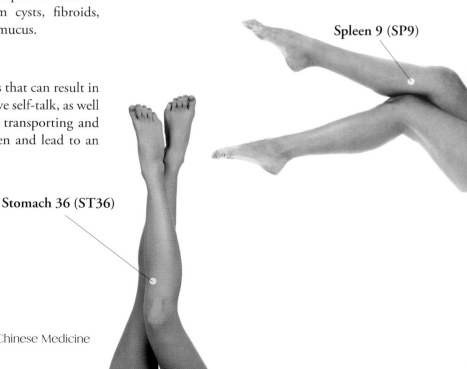

Spleen 9 (SP9)

Stomach 36 (ST36)

4: Blood Stagnation

- **Headache Pattern:** prolonged headaches, steady and stabbing pain, medications don't seem to help, often occurring in the same location, aggravated at night or during rainy days. This type is more common in older people and those with a history of a head injury. It can also be a result of injuries that have created Blood stagnation, which affect the head. The impaired Blood flow results in this pattern.

- **Accompanying Symptoms:** stroke, seizure disorder, dull and or darkish complexion, purple tongue, menstrual pain, vertigo, chronic tinnitus, hair loss, deafness, muscle weakness, sudden loss of vision. Blood stagnation also affects the Shen, causing insomnia (more on that on page 20).

HOW TO HEAL

- **Lifestyle:** A consistent, moderate exercise routine helps Blood and Qi to flow smoothly and not become stagnated. Anything that feels stuck, whether it be your emotions or body, can manifest in your body's flow as well. Qigong and stretching are also great practices for the flow of Blood and Qi.

- **Herbs:** Drink Ginger Power Tea (page 125) to invigorate Blood flow. Consume San Qi (page 135) to help circulation and Blood. Hawthorn berries are used as an herbal treatment in TCM and are known for their benefits for the Heart. Hawthorn has the ability to widen the vessels, increasing the amount of Blood pumped out from the Heart and increasing nerve signals responsible for smooth flow. It is used to treat coronary disease, hypertension, hyperlipidemia and Heart disease.

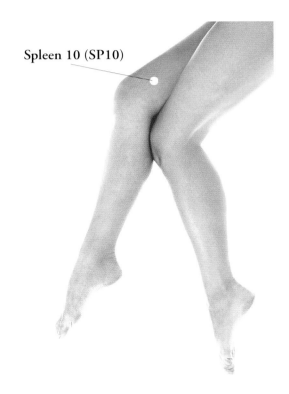

Spleen 10 (SP10)

- **Acupressure: Spleen 10** 血海 Xuehai is known as the "Sea of Blood" as it nourishes Blood and Qi. It's located with your knee flexed, 2 cun (2 finger widths) above the superior middle border of the kneecap on the bulge of the middle part of the quad. This is especially helpful to do at 10:30 a.m. Stimulate this point for 3 to 5 minutes on both legs.

5: Yin Deficiency

- **Headache Pattern:** Headaches that are accompanied with the below symptoms can be aggravated by going to bed late. This pattern is typically associated with aging or those in menopause.

- **Accompanying Symptoms:** aching low back and knees, red face, night sweats, hot flashes, infertility, impotence, vertigo, tinnitus, easily agitated, lethargy, restless sleep, dry stool, constipation, scanty urination, dry mouth, red tongue with less or no coating, palms of the hands could be hot, as well as soles of the feet.

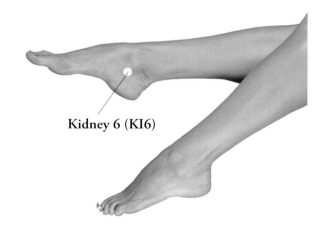

Kidney 6 (KI6)

HOW TO HEAL

- **Lifestyle:** Nourish Yin energy through meditation, stillness and self-reflection. Take time to slow down. Go to bed before 10:30 p.m. Soak feet one to seven nights a week in hot water (find a temperature that is manageable for you, don't burn yourself!) for 10 to 15 minutes to regulate heat. If you suffer from diabetes, please have someone test the temperature of the water so you don't burn yourself.

- **Foods:** Avoid alcohol, all spicy foods and hot sauces. Make sure to go to bed early and use meditation to replenish Yin.

- **Herbs:** Mulberries (page 134) and goji berries (page 133) support Yin greatly and can be taken daily.

- **Acupressure: Kidney 6** 照海 Zha Chai "Shining Sea" helps to nourish Yin. It is located in the depression below the tip of the medial malleolus—the bony bump on the inner side of the ankle. Apply pressure or rub for 2 to 3 minutes on both sides daily.

6: Kidney Yang Deficiency

- **Headache Pattern:** headaches with an emptiness sensation mostly at the crown of the head, aggravated by emotional distress and fatigue, and alleviated after sleeping, along with much aversion to cold.

- **Accompanying Symptoms:** pale face, dizziness, loose stool, blurred vision, cold body, cold hands and feet, fatigue, back and knee soreness, sweat easily, emission in those with a penis, white vaginal discharges, tinnitus, insomnia, forgetfulness, poor appetite.

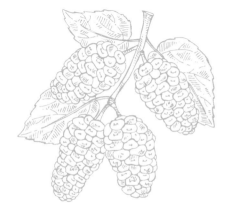

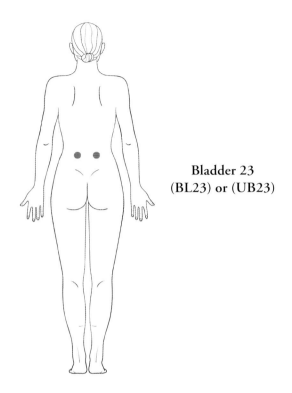

**Bladder 23
(BL23) or (UB23)**

HOW TO HEAL

• **Lifestyle:** Practice the key takeaways of the Kidney system (page 41) to boost Kidney function. Focus on dressing warmly. You can apply a heating pad to your lower back to help warm the area. Avoid overexertion with work, sex, partying and stress. These are specifically draining for the Kidney system. Practice moxibustion (page 74), which is burning the herb moxa close to the skin, on point **Bladder 23** 腎俞 "Sea of Vitality." This point is located at the waist on the lower back between the second and third lumbar vertebrae, two finger widths from the spine. If you would like to try this yourself, you can purchase moxa sticks online and ask a trusty friend to help you since the point is on the back. If you do not feel comfortable doing this, please do not do it at home and instead find a trusted practitioner.

• **Food:** If you eat meat, incorporate lamb into your diet twice weekly as it is very warming. Avoid anything cold, whether it be an iced beverage or exposing your Stomach.

• **Herb:** Ginger Power Tea (page 125) daily warms the body from the inside out.

7: Blood Deficiency

• **Headache Pattern:** dizziness, dull or pricking pain that is mostly in the temples.

• **Accompanying Symptoms:** migraine, pale and dull face and lips, irritability, a feverish sensation, thirst, hair loss, dry and brittle hair, palpitations, fatigue, poor memory, menstrual disorders like scanty period, general weakness, insomnia, emotional and/ or mental disharmonies.

HOW TO HEAL

• **Lifestyle:** Imbalanced emotions can cause Blood to become deficient, so finding ways to balance emotions naturally is important. This can be done through therapy, gratitude, volunteering, writing and creative expression.

• **Foods:** Learn how to build the Blood (page 23) and include more grass-fed red meat, Bone Broths (page 121) and dark leafy greens in your diet. Supplement with magnesium and beef liver pills that are now available at most health food stores and online. Make sure to eat a warming breakfast daily to boost digestive function to have better Blood flow.

• **Herbs:** I make a tincture called Blood Builder that features five of the most powerful herbs to boost the Blood. This is especially helpful for those who do not eat meat. This herbal formula is available on my website (lilychoinaturalhealing.com).

• **Acupressure:** Use the same point for Blood Stagnation: **Spleen 10** 血海 "Sea of Blood" (page 89).

8: External Pathogens Attack the Body

• **Headache Pattern:** pain felt in the back of the skull and/or the temple because of wind and or cold invading (these pathogens attack the upper part of the body), experienced after being exposed to wind or cold weather.

• **Accompanying Symptoms:** neck tightness or ache, runny nose, sneezing, itchy eyes, shoulder aches or soreness, fatigue.

HOW TO HEAL

• **Lifestyle:** Wear a scarf and dress warmly on the legs and neck to cover the essential meridians that run through those areas particularly. Wear socks during seasonal transitions or on colder and windier days. Take a warm bath with Epsom salts several times a week. This is a great way to cultivate internal warmth.

• **Foods:** Make Congee (page 114) and drink Bone Broth (page 121) daily to increase Qi.

• **Acupressure: Gallbladder 20** 風池 "Wind Pool" can be effective for many migraines, headaches, eye issues and that feeling like you just caught a cold. GB20 is located at the back of the head, at two points on both sides of the dip between the skull and the neck. The two points are to the left and the right of that dip in the neck. It will most likely feel tender there. Using your thumbs, hold your fingers on the points gently but with firm pressure for 1 minute. If the headache hasn't been relieved, continue holding the GB20 points until the headache starts to lift. Repeat as many times as needed at the onset of a headache.

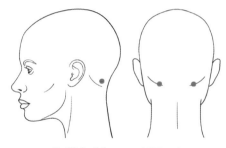

Gallbladder 20 (GB20)

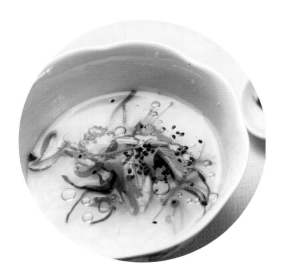

Insomnia

Two of my initial questions to every patient I treat are "What time do you go to bed?" and "How is your sleep?" The quality of your sleep is something you should always be taking inventory of, as it is indicative of what your body needs depending on your sleep patterns and habits.

Quality sleep is one of the pillars of health. I can't stress this enough: Sleep is one of the most overlooked healing tools. Think about how you feel after a good night's rest—renewed and nourished—compared to a poor night's sleep—agitated, fatigued and foggy. After a solid sleep, you are much more inclined to do all the things that make you feel good, like eat healthy and exercise. But without proper sleep, you may spend the day searching for comforts that are not necessarily benefiting your mental, physical or spiritual health.

What Causes This?

According to the Chinese medicine body clock, 11 p.m. begins the 2-hour window of Qi ruling in the Gallbladder (page 26). This is the ultimate transition time, the pivot from the waning of Yin to the emergence of Yang. This makes it the ideal time to be in bed asleep. The organs that are in focus at night are the Liver, then the Lung, then the Large Intestine. During each of these 2-hour windows of Qi, detoxification and regenerative processes occur. Like a store, it is easier to restock, clean and prepare for the next day after business hours when there's no one in the store and it is quiet.

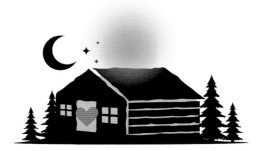

If the heart is unable to house the Shen, it will wander through the night causing insomnia.

Insomnia is a manifestation of a Shen disorder, which can usually fit into four major patterns. It is common to suffer from more than one pattern. Many of the patterns here are the same as the headache patterns (page 86) and treated the same way. This is a prime example of the same root cause manifesting in a different symptom dependent on the person.

The Four Insomnia Patterns and How to Heal Each

Insomnia Pattern 1

Emotional disturbance makes it difficult to fall and stay asleep. Excess heat or toxins in the Liver can stop the flow of emotions and cause imbalance, creating Liver Yang Rising (page 107). Symptoms include anger, stress, becoming easily agitated, nightmares, headache, red eyes, red tongue with red sides, bitter taste and dry mouth.

Insomnia (continued)

HOW TO HEAL

- **Emotions:** Calm the Liver. This is done through a variety of techniques, the largest being emotional balance. Stress, anger and frustration play a large role in this pattern of insomnia. Do you find yourself loosing sleep in a specific scenario or when you have a certain obligation? There is always an emotional connection. Bring your boundaries to match the needs of your body, as your body is signaling that there is a discord between your mind and your Heart. Write out your feelings daily, as you may not be expressing them fully.

- **Lifestyle:** Meditate daily and go to sleep before 11 p.m. Unplug from technology well before bed to allow your mind to peel back the layers from the day. What do you feel? Where do you feel it?

- **Acupressure:** Use your index and middle fingers to press and release on **Gallbladder 8** 率谷 "Valley Lead" on both sides. GB8 is located directly above the highest point of the ear, ½ inch (1.3 cm) from the top of the outside of the ear. Press and release quite vigorously on and around the point for three to five minutes as needed.

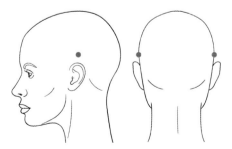

Gallbladder 8 (GB8)

Insomnia Pattern 2

Dampness can create nightmares and make it easy to wake up during the night. One of the Six Evils (page 46), this pathogen often manifests as a sluggish feeling, swelling and excess weight. Symptoms related to insomnia are chest and Stomach distension and thick yellow tongue coating. This pattern often manifests from eating an excess of greasy, heavy food, which in turn makes you crave those foods more.

HOW TO HEAL

- **Food:** Maintain proper eating habits and avoid skipping meals, especially breakfast. Refer to the warming foods and simple and bland diet (page 113). Avoid cold drinks, iced water or smoothies as they dim the digestive fire. Avoid dairy and sugars as you heal from this condition.

- **Acupressure:** **Spleen 9** 陰陵泉 "Yin Mound Spring" is located on the inside of the leg, under the knee in the soft spot just next to the border of the top of the tibia and calf muscle. By pressing on this point, on both legs, you can help open the channel to invigorate proper Blood and Qi flow, helping to relieve dampness (page 47) and its related symptoms. Do note that this point can be very tender when there are symptoms of dampness.

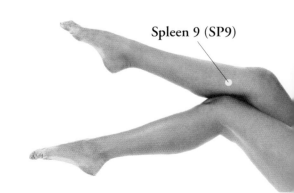

Spleen 9 (SP9)

Insomnia Pattern 3

Deficiency of the Spleen creates excessive dreams. You are easily awakened and unable to fall back asleep or wake up early. When the Spleen is deficient and unable to transmit and assimilate food and nutrients properly, it loses its smooth connection to the Heart. Symptoms can include palpitations; dizzy, blurred vision; fatigue; overthinking and worrying; and poor memory. The Spleen and the Heart need to be connected with proper Blood flow in order to keep this connection strong.

HOW TO HEAL

• **Food:** Commit to regular eating with healthy food choices and avoid too much raw and cold food. Boost the energy of the Spleen with ginger, red dates, cinnamon and warm water.

• **Lifestyle:** Reduce overworking and avoid over-thinking, which improperly spends too much precious digestive energy. If you have a habit of not setting proper emotional boundaries, it can contribute to Spleen deficiency.

Insomnia Pattern 4

Disconnection of the Kidney and the Heart result in difficulty falling asleep. Kidneys don't have enough energy to support the digestion to nourish the Heart. This nourishing mist is the energy the Spleen transmits from the food we eat. Symptoms include fear, irritability, restlessness, severe continuous palpitations, cold feet, high blood sugar, loose stool, headaches, tinnitus, dry mouth and back pain.

HOW TO HEAL

• **Food:** Avoid all spicy foods and hot sauces. Refrain from drinking alcohol during this period.

• **Lifestyle:** Nourish Yin energy through Qigong (page 55), meditation, stillness and self-reflection. Take time to slow down and unwind as the sun sets. This practice directly connects you to the Yin part of the day in order to nourish yours. Go to bed before 10:30 p.m. Soak feet one to seven nights a week in hot water (find a temperature that is manageable for you, don't burn yourself!) for 10 to 15 minutes in order to regulate heat. If you suffer from diabetes, please have someone test the temperature of the water for you so you don't burn yourself.

• **Herbs:** Insomnia IV is a tincture I make specifically to connect the Kidney and the Heart for this imbalance. It is available on my website (lilychoinaturalhealing.com).

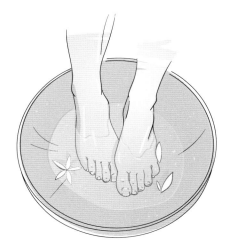

Memory Loss

Several underlying causes can bring about memory problems. According to Western medicine, forgetfulness and memory problems can arise from stress, depression, lack of sleep, thyroid problems, certain medicines, an unhealthy diet or not having enough fluids in your body. This can all be very well true, but there is an even deeper connection and way to make sure memory stays strong. I have noticed that even my younger patients are complaining about poor memory or cognitive function.

What Causes This?

In TCM, there are several factors that can contribute to the feeling of poor memory or forgetfulness. A healthy mind involves harmony between the Sea of Marrow, also known as the Brain, and the Shen (page 20), which is the spirit ruled by the Heart. Our memory is most influenced by the Spleen, the Kidney and the Heart organ systems. If they are experiencing an imbalance or deficiency, it can very well spill over into brain dysfunction.

How Do Certain Organ Systems Play a Role in Memory?

• **Spleen** influences short-term memory, analytical thinking, studying, memorizing, focusing, generating ideas and concentration. It is damaged by improper nutrition and worrying too much. The Chinese word for the mental aspect of the Spleen is "Yi," which can be translated to idea or intention.

• **Heart** is for long-term memory and recall. It is damaged by emotional and chemical overstimulation. The Heart controls Blood: If there is dysfunction in this organ system, the Blood won't receive proper nourishment. The Heart and the Spleen both play an integral role in the quality, quantity and movement of Blood.

• **Kidney** dictates short-term memory and retention. It is damaged by fear and aging, which is essentially the loss of Jing (page 20), our essence that supplies the body with the energy in charge of adrenals, hormone balance and genetics received from your conception.

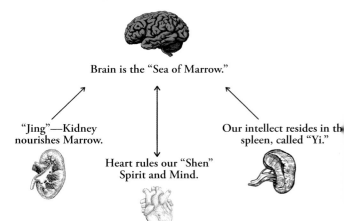

Brain is the "Sea of Marrow."

"Jing"—Kidney nourishes Marrow.

Heart rules our "Shen" Spirit and Mind.

Our intellect resides in the spleen, called "Yi."

How to Heal

Foods and Herbs

• Rou Cong-Rong 肉鬆蓉 or Herba Cistanche, commonly known as "desert ginseng," is one of the best pharmaceutical gifts of TCM because it strengthens precious Yang energy and the Kidney system, as well as cognitive function.[1]

• Ginkgo biloba is widely touted as a "brain herb" and has been noted to improve memory loss associated with Blood circulation abnormalities.

• Magnesium L-threonate has shown great promise for cognitive function. Studies in animals and humans show that magnesium L-threonate improves and maintains cognitive function, even in older individuals with prior signs of cognitive decline. In one human study, it reversed cognitive measures of brain aging by 9 years.[2]

---

1   Li Zhiming et al., "Herba Cistanche (Rou Cong-Rong): One of the Best Pharmaceutical Gifts of Traditional Chinese Medicine," *Frontiers in Pharmacology* 7, no. 41 (2016): 10.3389/fphar.2016.00041
2   Stein Harry, "Magnesium L-Threonate Regenerates Brain Structures," *Life Extension* (2022): www.lifeextension.com/magazine/2020/6/magnesium-l-threonate-regenerates-brain-structures

Acupressure

• **Pericardium 8 or PC 8** 勞宮 "Palace of Toil" is a point on the Pericardium meridian (page 42), which is like the Heart protector. This point helps memory, Alzheimer's disease and easing the mind. If you make a fist, it is located about where the middle fingertip touches the palm. Like the motion of rubbing your hands together to warm them, keep going to bring your hand over the other hands' fingers and squeeze them. When you squeeze your fingers, you will notice that you are stimulating point PC 8. Do this motion as fast as you can for about 6 to 7 minutes. Practice several times per day. This exercise is said to brighten the brain.

• Find the tender spot right in the center of the top of the head. Stimulate this point and the four points that can be found 1 inch (2.5 cm) away from the center in each direction: right, left, front and back. Do this by applying gentle but deep, downward pressure with your finger to each of these five points, 50 to 60 times each day.

• Massage the ears. Gently knead the whole outer ear, especially the earlobe, until it is warm and red. This will stimulate many beneficial acupressure points located on the ear and nourish the Kidneys.

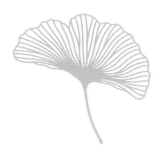

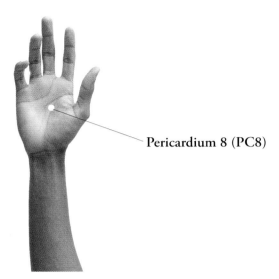

Pericardium 8 (PC8)

Menopause

Menopause is when a woman has gone without a menstrual period for 12 consecutive months. At this stage, the ovaries have stopped releasing eggs and producing most of their estrogen.

Menopause is another stage in a woman's development, one that should be nearly asymptomatic. From what I've seen in my practice over the years, this is far from the case. Researchers from the Department of Integrated Health at Westminster University polled 1,000 British women ages 45 to 55 and compared their answers to those of women from the United States, Canada, Japan and China. The conclusion was that Japanese and Chinese women suffer the least amount of menopause symptoms, British women suffer the most and Americans are close behind.[1]

---

1   Scheid Volker et al., "Chinese medicine treatment for menopausal symptoms in the UK health service: is a clinical trial warranted?," *Maturitas* 80, no. 2 (2015): 179-186, 10.1016/j.maturitas.2014.11.006

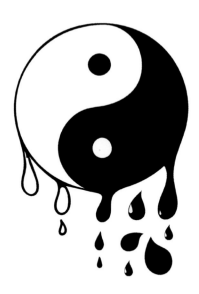

What Causes This?

In TCM, we say that menopause is when a woman stops "wasting Blood." Blood can now nourish her Heart and allow her to embrace her wisdom and role as a leader in her family and community.

TCM categorizes menopause as Kidney Yin deficiency and includes symptoms like gray hair and ending menstruation. These are signs of reduced Kidney energy, which is natural as we age. When there is an imbalance of Kidney Yin and Yang, however, symptoms such as hot flashes, insomnia and night sweats arise. Through balancing the body's internal thermostat, the Yin (cool) and Yang (heat), we can ease these symptoms. Although many women feel symptoms of too much heat, it is a result of too low Yin energy or fluids, which makes the body dry and hot. I like to refer to this as artificial heat.

How to Heal

Foods and Herbs

• Nourish Yang with Ginger Power Tea (page 125) daily before 6 p.m.

• Schisandra (page 136) is a beloved herb of TCM, which denotes all five taste senses at once. It is especially helpful for the Liver and the Kidney systems and treats menopausal symptoms stemming from Kidney Qi deficiency, including profuse sweating, night sweats and frequent urination. Schisandra balances Kidney fluids and overall strengthens Kidney Qi. A 2016 study analyzed the effects of schisandra extract on women with menopausal symptoms, following thirty-six menopausal women for one year. Researchers determined that schisandra is effective at alleviating some symptoms of menopause like hot flashes, sweating and heart palpitations.[2]

2   Park J Y and Kim K H, "A randomized, double-blind, placebo-controlled trial of Schisandra chinensis for menopausal symptoms," *Climacteric* 19, no. 6 (2016): 574-580, 10.1080/13697137.2016.1238453

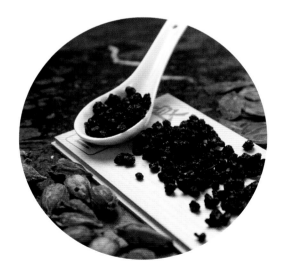

• Incorporate daily the five flavors of salty, bitter, sour, pungent and sweet into your diet to nourish all organ systems. Avoid spicy foods in the forms of hot sauces and spicy peppers. For the pungent category, focus more on scallions, ginger and garlic.

• Other herbal support can be found from goji berries (page 133), Du Zhong (page 131) and mulberries (page 134).

• Enjoy wild yams, sweet potatoes, black beans, snow mushroom, black wood ear mushroom, dates, bitter melon, lotus root, pears and organic non-GMO soy.

• Add a few foods that are categorized as having a "cooling" effect on the body to help internal air-conditioning. These are foods like daikon radishes, mung beans, dandelion greens, bok choy, kale, celery and asparagus—but make sure they are all cooked (read more on the importance of that on page 117).

• Avoid alcohol consumption. Depending on where you are on your menopause journey, alcohol can exacerbate symptoms such as hot flashes, mood swings and insomnia.

Lifestyle

• Nourish Yin through daily meditation and an early bedtime. Go to bed before 11 p.m.

• Embrace this new chapter of your life and remember it is all about perspective.

Men's Fertility

It takes three months for your body to produce mature sperm. During this time, TCM methods used alongside proper diet and lifestyle habits can successfully create balance and enhance fertility.

What Causes This?

Male infertility can be traced and treated through the Kidney system. The main cause of infertility in men is the result of Kidney deficiency. The reason the Kidney is so vital in both male and female fertility is because this organ is the supplier of Yin and Yang for all other organs, while also being the base for birth, growth and reproduction. The Kidney organ system also stores Jing 精 (page 38), the essential fluid of our physical body that defines our basic constitution, with similarities to our DNA.

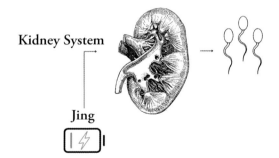

How to Heal

Food and Herbs

• A diet rich in nourishing and nutritious whole foods like almonds, anchovies, avocados, black beans, black sesame seeds, Brussels sprouts, Bone Broth (page 121), chicken, coconut, dark leafy greens, eggs, fish, ghee, kidney beans, mung beans, mussels, organ meats, oysters, raspberries, salmon, sardines, sea weeds, sea salt and wheat grass. Do note that all foods, especially animal products, are best as organic and sustainable when possible.

• Foods to avoid, as they harm the reproductive system, include alcohol, an excess of cold or raw foods, foods you find difficult to digest, processed foods, spicy foods, refined sugars, excess salt and sodium.

• He Shou Wu (何首烏) is a popular remedy that is derived from the fo-ti (Polygonum multiflorum) plant. This herb supports and strengthens not only the Kidney organ system but also the Liver organ system, helping to support fertility. This herb is the main ingredient in my tincture called Follicle Power, which is available on my website (lilychoinatural-healing.com).

Lifestyle

• Choose moderate and consistent exercise as opposed to constant strenuous activities where lots of sweat occurs.

• Look into receiving acupuncture to open meridians and unblock any stagnation in the body.

• Manage emotions and stress. Take time to unwind naturally, without drugs or drinking.

• Activities to avoid when trying to conceive are hot baths, hot tubs, eating late at night, overeating, saunas, smoking, drug use and placing your computer, cellphone and iPad on your lap or in your pants pocket.

Osteoporosis

Osteoporosis is a bone disease that occurs when the body loses too much bone, makes too little bone or both. As a result, bones become weak and may break from a fall or, in serious cases, from something minor. The body constantly absorbs and replaces bone tissue, but with osteoporosis, new bone creation doesn't keep up with old bone removal.

What Causes This?

In TCM, the Kidney system stores our inherited "essence" we call Jing (page 38). Jing is responsible for promoting the growth and repair of marrow, which nourishes the bones and strengthens them. When Kidney deficiency is present, it can decrease estrogen levels, leading to osteoporosis. This explains why postmenopausal women are susceptible—the drop of estrogen leads to more bone resorption than formation, resulting in osteoporosis.[1]

How to Heal

Foods and Herbs

• Have Ginger Power Tea (page 125) daily before 6 p.m. to nourish the Spleen in order to support all the other organ systems.

• Du Zhong (page 131) is an herb that helps strengthen weak legs and the back, tonifies the Liver and the Kidney systems and strengthens tendons and bones.

• Have 1 tablespoon (9 g) of black sesame seeds daily, freshly ground for optimal absorption, or use my Black Sesame Seed Extract tincture available on my website (lilychoinaturalhealing.com).

• Schisandra (page 136) helps regulate hormones through the Kidney and the Liver channels.

• Supplement with magnesium and vitamin D3.

• Remove all sugars and refined carbohydrates from your diet.

Lifestyle

• Strength training or weightlifting has been shown to help protect bones, prevent osteoporosis-related fractures, prevent bone loss and may even help build new bone.

• Tap the teeth to help strengthen the Kidney system! Read more about this practice on page 41.

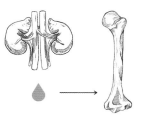

"Jing"—Kidney Essence nourishes Marrow.

1   Ji Meng-Xia and Yu Qi, "Primary osteoporosis in postmenopausal women," *Chronic Diseases and Translational Medicine* 1, no. 1 (2015): 9-13, 10.1016/j. cdtm.2015.02.006

Painful Periods

A menstruating person is given a gift every month: their period. This gift allows physical and emotional detoxification. Unfortunately, because of the physical and emotional toll an imbalanced period takes on the modern person, this time of the month is often seen as less of a gift and more of a curse.

What Causes This?

Teens may experience a bit of premenstrual syndrome and cramps during their period. If they learn some general tips on how to take care of themselves, they can regulate to a normal cycle early on. If not—and if they develop a lifestyle that includes overworking, poor diet, worry and strenuous exercise—they may find themselves in more pain when their period comes as they get older.

Years of these symptoms can lead to conditions like infertility and severe menstrual imbalances. Does this sound familiar? Do you wish you knew a bit earlier these conditions around menstruation that are labeled normal—bloating, breast tenderness, headaches, mood swings and painful and irregular periods—are actually not considered normal according to TCM?

With consistent natural lifestyle practices, taking emotional inventory and connecting to the natural rhythm of your body (i.e., rest when necessary), you can connect to the gift that the period really provides.

Continued long-term use of modern hormonal methods of contraception create a negative impact on hormones and fertility. Birth control specifically suppresses the healthy functioning of the Liver.

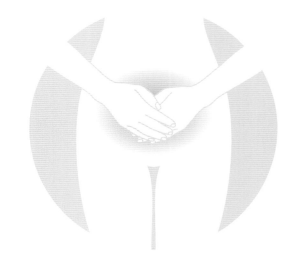

How to Heal

Foods and Herbs

• Eat warming breakfast daily (page 113).

• According to ancient Chinese medicine texts, "During a menstrual cycle, one should avoid spicy and fried foods, as these foods may cause heatiness," and emotional or physical reactions associated with temper and excess.

• Avoid cold and raw foods just prior to and during menstruation.

Lifestyle

• Just prior to and during menstruation, people should consider their emotions and not worry or dwell on bothersome thoughts. Avoid the following just prior to and during menstruation: vigorous exercise, intensive stress and sex. Sex reverses the flow of Qi and Blood from down and out to up and in and tends to cause the formation of Blood stagnation.

Acupressure

• **Spleen 6** 三陰交 "Three Yin Intersection" is one of the most beneficial points for menstruation, reproduction and menopause. This is because SP6 is the intersection point of the Spleen, the Kidney and the Liver systems, which are the three major organs governing the menstrual cycle and hormones. This point is roughly four finger widths from the bony bump on the inner side of the ankle. If it is comfortable, you can press the point on both ankles by getting into a modified cross-legged position. If that doesn't work for you, just press one side at a time by sitting upright with your ankle crossed over your opposite leg. Using your hand on the same side as the leg you are pressing, come from above the point and place your thumb at SP6. Grasping your leg with your fingers, apply firm pressure with your thumb for 2 to 3 minutes daily. *Do not use this point during pregnancy, as this is one of the main points we use to help induce labor.*

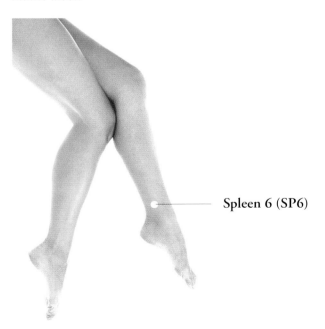

Spleen 6 (SP6)

Stress

Stress is the body's natural reaction to pressure, challenge or demand that results in emotional and/or physical tension. In small doses, low-degree and short-term stress can be positive to finish an assignment or defend your body from a dangerous situation, because this lets the body practice protecting itself. But now more than ever, our on-the-go lifestyle and constant connection results in an excess of stressful situations. When stress builds up, it can lead to health problems.

So many people tell me, "I went to the doctor, all my tests came back normal, but I still feel all these symptoms and don't feel well." Just because something doesn't show up on a scan or a blood test does not mean you are not suffering or don't have a problem. The symptom itself is signaling that there is something wrong.

What Causes This?

Stress can affect all organs and systems in the body, beginning in the central nervous system and the endocrine system. These systems receive an alert that action needs to take place and the brain alerts the body to produce cortisol and adrenaline (hormones to help us manage the stressors). Prolonged stress keeps the body in this protective mode and eventually exhausts the systems little by little. High blood pressure, chronic fatigue, hypertension, autoimmune conditions and even risk of heart attack or stroke can follow.

The Liver oversees the regulation of our emotions and the circulation our vital life force energy, Qi. The Spleen governs the digestive system and is supported by the Liver, as the smooth flow of Qi is essential for the smooth circulation of Blood throughout the digestive system. If this flow is not harmonious and if the Liver is experiencing dysfunction, it is unable to support the Spleen and can even attack it, causing weak digestion.

A recent study found that high levels of stress can affect gut bacteria similarly to a high-fat diet, while other studies have shown that reducing the number of bacteria in the gut can produce stress-induced activity in mice.[1]

A Closer Look at Root Cause Symptoms

• **Liver Qi Stagnation:** feeling gloomy or easily angered, pain or distension in the chest and/or ribs, frequent sighing, feeling restless.

• **Spleen Deficiency:** poor appetite, stomach bloating, chronic fatigue, loose stools, flatulence.

---

1 Madison Annelise and Kiecolt-Glaser Janice K, "Stress, depression, diet, and the gut microbiota: human-bacteria interactions at the core of psychoneuroimmunology and nutrition," *Current Opinion in Behavioral Sciences* 28, (2019): 105-110, 10.1016/j.cobeha.2019.01.011

How to Heal

Foods and Herbs

• Calming and Cooling Tea (page 128) helps to calm the Liver to support stress relief.

Acupressure

• **Liver 3** Tai Chong 太衝 "Great Surge" is an incredible point for stress relief, emotional regulation, menstrual imbalance, eye issues and digestive disorders. You can easily find this point in the web at the top of the groove between the first and second toes. Pinch this point with your thumb and index finger or stimulate it while sitting in a chair with the heel of your opposite foot. You can do this throughout the day while you are sitting at your desk. Practice for 2 to 3 minutes on both feet daily.

Liver 3 (LV3)

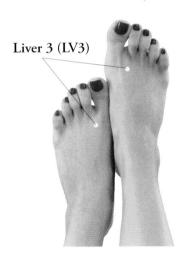

• Rub the ribs! There are some influential points of the Liver meridian (page 42) that run through the rib cage. Through stimulating them, you can invigorate, as well as relieve, the Liver. Sit or stand upright with your feet shoulder-width apart. Place the palm of the left hand on the left ribcage area and the palm of the right hand on the right ribcage area. Move both hands back and forth in a rubbing motion for 10 seconds, rest and repeat for another 10 seconds. Perform this exercise two to three times a day.

Lifestyle

• Exercise and movement help to unblock the flow of Qi and Blood, a.k.a. reduce stagnation, while minimizing the effects of stress on our mind and body. Tai Chi, yoga, Qigong (page 55) and stretching or forms of exercise that focus on breathing and meditation further help to move Qi.

• Walking, connecting to our natural environment and moving our body simultaneously has its benefits. Recent studies have documented that time in nature, as long as people feel safe, is an antidote for stress. It can lower Blood pressure and stress hormone levels, reduce nervous system arousal, enhance immune system function, increase self-esteem, reduce anxiety and improve mood.[2]

---

2   Robbins Jim, "Ecopsychology: How Immersion in Nature Benefits Your Health," *Yale Environment* 360, (2020): yale.edu/features/ecopsychology-how-immersion-in-nature-benefits-your-health

Tinnitus

If you suffer from tinnitus, your head is filled with sound—ringing, whistling, clicking and roaring—that no one else hears. This ringing or buzzing noise in one or both ears may be constant or come and go. It can be associated with hearing loss at its worst.

According to Western medicine, tinnitus results from underlying conditions, such as age-related hearing loss, an ear injury or a problem with the circulatory system. This is aligned with TCM as well, as tinnitus and ear-ringing are symptoms but not necessarily conditions.

Similar to headaches (page 86) and insomnia (page 93), there are different patterns of tinnitus in TCM.

What Causes This?

In TCM, the ears are a manifestation of the Kidney system and we say that the Kidney opens to the ears. There are two main causes that manifest into tinnitus symptoms: excess and deficient types. Excess is easier to treat, while deficient is more chronic and lingering. Both are treatable, but the deficient type does takes more time.

For example, in more temporary cases of tinnitus, high emotional strain or sudden anger can lead to a ringing in the ears. Also, diet can have an effect. Excessive greasy foods or irregular eating can lead to dampness (page 47) and retention in body fluid, which prevents the rising of clear Qi to the head, resulting in the "phantom noise" associated with tinnitus. For more lasting cases, overworking or excessive physical strain can lead to a nerve disturbance, causing tinnitus. Lastly, trauma is a common cause of the ringing noise associated with this disorder.

Before we dive in, whichever pattern you most associate with in the following section, here are some healing modalities that help with symptoms from all types: Perform acupressure on **Small Intestine 19** 聽宮 Ting Gong "Hearing Palace." It is on the Small Intestine channel. This point specifically can release dampness and phlegm accumulation, which often is the root cause of tinnitus and vertigo. Sit properly and open your mouth in order to locate the point and feel the depression by the ear. Place your thumb or index finger at the point with the mouth still open and gently massage in a small circle for 1 to 3 minutes once daily. Repeat on both sides. Drink a cup of warm water or Ginger Power Tea (page 125) afterward.

Small Intestine 19 (SI19)

The Two Patterns of Tinnitus and How to Heal Each

1. Excess

LIVER YANG RISING

Emotions cause symptoms such as big wave or storm-like sounds, sounds coming on suddenly, loud or high-pitched sounds, sounds that are stronger when angry or agitated and ear pain. Associated symptoms can be headaches, dizziness, red face, red eyes, bitter mouth, dry throat, lack of sound sleep, rib pain, constipation, yellow urine, red tongue with yellow coating or a wiry strong pulse. This is due to emotions, trauma, stress and/or lifestyle.

HOW TO HEAL

• **Lifestyle:** Go to bed before 11 p.m. Use meditation and natural stress relief methods.
• **Foods:** Avoid spicy and/or greasy foods.

DAMPNESS OBSTRUCTION

Weak Spleen function creates dampness. This type can be constant ringing, which can even affect hearing. Associated symptoms may include you not being able to hear clearly or your head feeling heavy, light headaches, chest tightness, coughing with lots of phlegm, constipation, greasy tongue and slippery pulse. This is mostly due to diet.

HOW TO HEAL

• **Foods:** Avoid dairy, gluten, inflammatory foods, refined sugars, and cold and greasy foods.

WIND HEAT

An invasion of the external pathogens wind and heat disrupt the Triple Warmer meridian (page 42). Sudden onset of ringing lasts temporarily. Associated symptoms alternate between chill and fever.

HOW TO HEAL

• **Foods and Herbs:** Eat mung beans and lentils. Incorporate cooling herbs like Self-Heal (page 137).
• **Acupressure:** Press **GB20** to remove wind. Massage for 2 to 3 minutes twice daily.

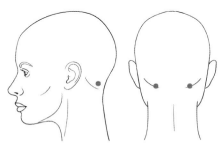

Gallbladder 20 (GB20)

2. Deficient

KIDNEY DEFICIENCY

This is usually the case for those over 45 years old or those dealing with menopause. This type is usually chronic, can lead to ringing all the time, low-pitched sound, and ringing sound that goes from light to strong. Associated symptoms can be difficulty hearing, dizziness, blurred vision, sore back and knees, hot flashes, dry stool and scanty urination.

HOW TO HEAL

• **Lifestyle:** Strengthen the Kidney system (page 38).

Vertigo

Vertigo is defined as a sudden internal or external spinning sensation, often triggered by moving your head too quickly. Vertigo and dizziness are symptoms but not necessarily conditions.

In TCM, the earliest mention of the term "vertigo" (眩暈) was discovered in an ancient medical text that stated, "諸風掉眩 皆屬於肝," which translates to "when the eyes are blurred and there is wind, the causes of vertigo are most likely related to the liver." The 眩 character denotes blurry eyes and the character 暈 expresses a spinning head.

What Causes This?

Next are the three main patterns that can result in vertigo in TCM. One or more root causes can occur at once. Vertigo can also be a result of an injury or trauma to the head.

Before we dive in, here are some healing methods that can help all patterns of vertigo. Supplement with magnesium, as there is a link with low magnesium levels and vertigo. Try regular chiropractic and acupuncture treatments. Perform acupressure on point **SP6** and **GB20**.

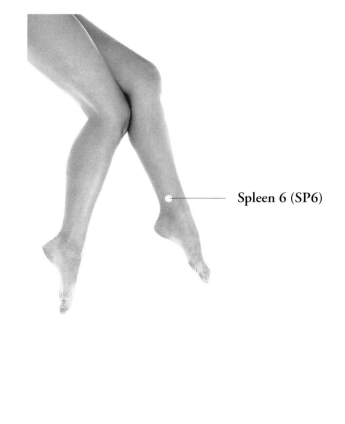

Spleen 6 (SP6)

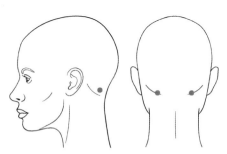

Gallbladder 20 (GB20)

The Three Patterns of Vertigo and How to Heal Each

Liver Yang Rising

Consistently experiencing emotional disturbances like anger, depression, frustration and even feeling like you're stuck in life damage Liver Yin and cause the rise of wind of Liver Yang to the top of the head.

HOW TO HEAL

•   **Lifestyle:** Strengthening and supporting the Liver (page 26) will help to balance emotions and the organ system. Make sure to get quality rest, which entails going to bed before 11 p.m. and avoiding screens about 2 hours before bed. Use your creativity, express yourself and speak your mind. If you find yourself getting angry, take a pause and be honest with yourself on why you are feeling this way without blaming others.

•   **Foods:** Don't eat late at night and don't skip breakfast. Avoid greasy, spicy foods.

Dampness

As one of the Six Evils (page 46), dampness (page 47) results from a weak digestion. A poor diet and an overconsumption of cold foods, cold drinks and raw foods can create dampness in the Spleen, phlegm and an overall heaviness. Fatigue and excess weight may also be symptoms. Feeling heavy and nauseous, in addition to the ringing of tinnitus, can indicate this is the root cause.

HOW TO HEAL

•   **Lifestyle:** Strengthen the Spleen (page 33). Engage in nourishing activities like walks in the park, stretching and Qigong movements (page 55).

•   **Food and Herbs:** Avoid cold drinks, raw foods, dairy, refined sugars and carbohydrates. Use warming foods like Ginger Power Tea (page 125), turmeric and black peppercorn.

Kidney Yang Deficiency

This pattern is like "burning the candle at both ends," so to speak. Aging, overwork and overexertion, drug use and overall exhaustion can lead to the early drainage of our life essence that we call Jing (page 20). In addition to your vertigo symptoms, other indicators of this root cause can be hair loss, early graying, fertility problems, body feeling cold, edema on legs, weak back and knees and joint pain.

HOW TO HEAL

•   **Lifestyle:** Nourish the Kidney system (page 38). Practice moxibustion (page 74). Remember to either have a professional do this for you or take extra care and precaution if performing this on yourself.

Women's Infertility

Infertility can be a frustrating and hard topic for many to discuss. If you feel like you've been running in circles and are starting to feel hopeless about conceiving, the next section can show you alternative ways to improve this personal matter. There are many herbal and naturopathic conversations popping up around infertility, but TCM has been understanding and healing infertility in women for centuries. For those going through in vitro fertilization, clinical research shows a 50 percent increase in fertility success rate with patients who underwent acupuncture than those who didn't in a controlled group study.[1]

---

1   Paulus Wolfgang E et al., "Influence of acupuncture on the pregnancy rate in patients who undergo assisted reproduction therapy," *Fertility and Sterility* 77, no. 4 (2002): 721-724, 10.1016/s0015-0282(01)03273-3

What Causes This?

Let's first understand fertility in TCM. Within each human there is Yin and Yang or Blood and Qi. In men, the reigning substance is Qi and for women it is Blood. When the Qi from Heaven (Yang) moves into the Blood of Earth (Yin), a new form of life begins. The force and action of this movement is ruled by Yang, but the receptive ability and essence required for nourishment is Yin. Their merger forms a new life. This is another showcase of Yang within Yin—the Yang then keeps the Yin warm, while the Yin nurtures.

Fertility is the natural expression of a body full of free-flowing and unobstructed Qi (life force) and Blood. Fertility treatment in TCM is like tending to your garden. You must prep the soil, nourish it and irrigate it properly for the chance of a seed to grow. Take three months to work on regulating your menstrual cycle prior to trying to conceive.

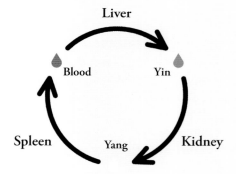

The three organ systems that work in synergy for conception

Liver

Blood — Yin

Spleen — Yang — Kidney

How to Heal

Foods and Herbs

• Healthy conception begins in the gut. A healthy Stomach and Spleen support the functioning of the reproductive organs. Eat a warming breakfast (page 113) and ditch the smoothies, salads and cold breakfast bowls. The uterus requires warmth for Blood and Qi to smoothly and freely flow and that warmth is generated in the digestive system. Iced drinks, salads and even leftovers use more vital energy because they need to be warmed up by the body before digested. The more these substances can move without stagnation, the easier it will be to conceive. Do not drink cold water or any ice-cold drinks during this time.

• Ample and free-flowing Blood is an integral part of fertility. Strengthen and build Blood with foods like Bone Broth (page 121), dark leafy greens, spirulina, seaweed soups, Congee (page 114), prunes, red dates, beets and black wood ear mushrooms.

• Organ meats provide us with the most digestible and usable form of vitamins and minerals. Grass-fed beef liver is a premium source of vitamins C, D, E and CoQ10, as well as zinc, folate and fat, all of which have been shown to play crucial roles in male and female fertility. It also is filled with B vitamins, which convert food energy into chemical energy for your cells. It is important to note that the only usable form of vitamin B-12 is found in animal foods, ideally wild-caught, grass-fed and/or pastured animal foods. In TCM, beef liver is known for its ability to tonify or strengthen Blood. For the best quality, I would go to your local farmers market and source organic, grass-fed and finished beef liver. You can also supplement with beef liver capsules available at your local health food store or online.

• Other notable foods are walnuts, wild salmon, sardines, oysters, black beans, adzuki beans, free-range eggs, sweet potatoes and wild yams.

Lifestyle

• Warm the body by covering crucial reproductive meridians. These include the belly, feet and ankles. Don't expose the Stomach or wear socks that come lower than the ankle if the weather is still cool, as this disrupts Blood flow.

• Substitute high-intensity exercise with slower-paced, mind-body connection activities like yoga, Qigong (page 55), Pilates, stretching and walks in nature. Intense exercise uses too much Qi, can cause inflammation and takes away Blood and Qi. Instead, use moderate exercise to balance energy gained and spent.

• Monitor your stress levels. One of the most common yet overlooked problems inhibiting conception is the umbrella of stress. This includes physical, emotional and environmental stress. The Liver is the organ system most affected by stress. When stressed, it attacks the Spleen, which is why one's appetite can fluctuate when stressed.

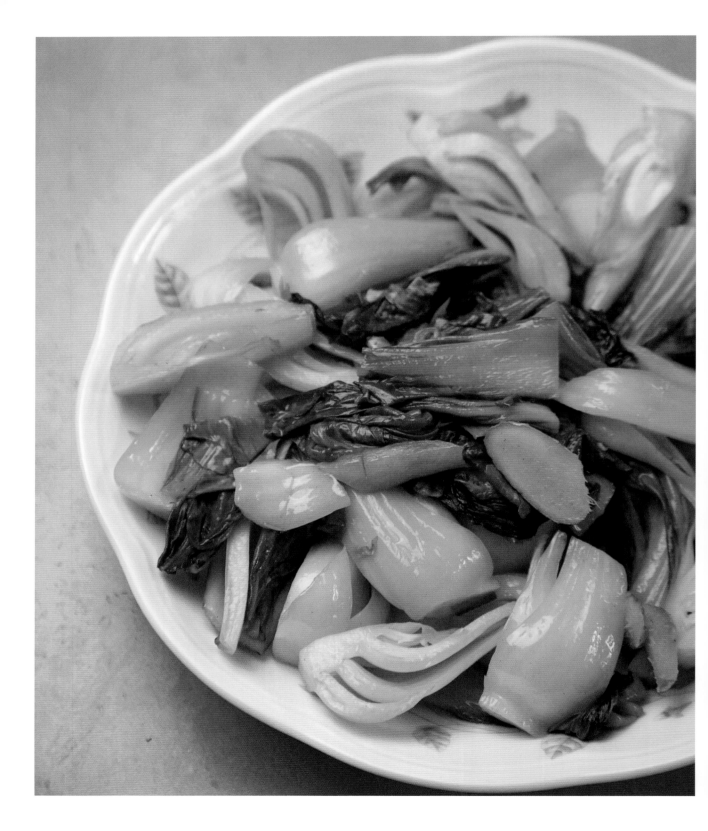

Chapter 6

Recipes and Herbal Formulas for Total Body Wellness

Throughout this book, we have talked about the importance of diet and how a poor diet can be the root cause of so many illnesses, chronic pains, discomforts and ailments. Now, I will teach you some of my favorite recipes, teas and herbal formulas that combat these issues and put the pillars of TCM to use.

We've also talked a great deal about how warming foods! 清淡 *translates to "Light and Simple Diet," which is a way of life, one utilized to harmonize the organs to their natural state of balance. Simple and light foods consist of vegetables and natural grains and have evolved to include broths, Bone Broths (page 121), soups, porridges and Congee (page 114), and proteins. This way of eating is believed to prevent diseases, strengthen the body and prolong life. Through hundreds of years of research and practice, the ancients concluded that such foods aid in resisting disease.*

What hurts the body? The consumption of heavy, greasy and sweet foods over a long period of time. These foods directly impact the Stomach, the Spleen and the Liver, and produce heat, phlegm and dampness (page 47). The Nei Jing says, "Heavy and greasy food causes a change that may result in serious illness." With that, let's dive into some of the recipes and formulas I've recommended throughout the book. These are some of the most powerful and useful tools for healing.

Congee

In Chinese, rice is translated to the character 米. The word Qi is 氣. As you can see, the 米 symbol is the foundation of the word Qi, so rice gives way to Qi.

The essence of this grain has long been used to heal people who suffer from Qi deficiency in the Spleen. This symptom can relate to a slow metabolism, excess body weight, leaky gut syndrome, premenstrual syndrome symptoms, food allergies, irritable bowel syndrome and other digestion disorders. For those reasons, rice is consumed first thing in the morning for breakfast as congee (粥). It warms the stomach and kick-starts the digestive system. Rice also cures stomachaches!

Did you know that your digestive system craves moist foods in the morning? The Spleen and the Stomach are most active between 7 and 11 a.m., when they are most nourished by moist, sweet (meaning certain grains, not refined sugars) and warm foods. That's what makes congee a healing breakfast, because it is able to be easily digested for usable energy.

Not limited to China, most cultures have their own version of a slow-cooked porridge for very good reason. Congee benefits hydration, gut health, lactation, postpartum symptoms and immunity. It improves digestive function to benefit the whole body through building Qi and Blood.

Here is an easy way to make one serving. This yields about ¾ cup (140 g) of cooked rice, so if you are worried about having too much rice, this makes just enough and will not spike your blood sugar.

Makes 1 serving

1 tbsp (13 g) uncooked rice

2 cups (480 ml) water or broth

Optional additions: minced meat, fish, salt or toppings of choice

On high in an uncovered pot, boil the rice in the water for about 10 minutes, stirring occasionally. Turn off the heat and cover for 30 minutes.

Uncover the pot and bring the heat to a medium-high flame to boil the rice again. Stir occasionally, and once it begins to bubble, you can lower the heat. If you want to add any minced meat or fish to your congee, add it now. Watch it carefully, as it should only be another 5 to 7 minutes before it's ready. The rice will begin to have a sticky and creamy consistency and that's when it will be done. This is the most important step, as that is where the healing lies!

Add a pinch of salt if you like or whatever toppings you are craving. The key is to get the right consistency. It is said that the stickiness is the most valuable part of congee for the Stomach!

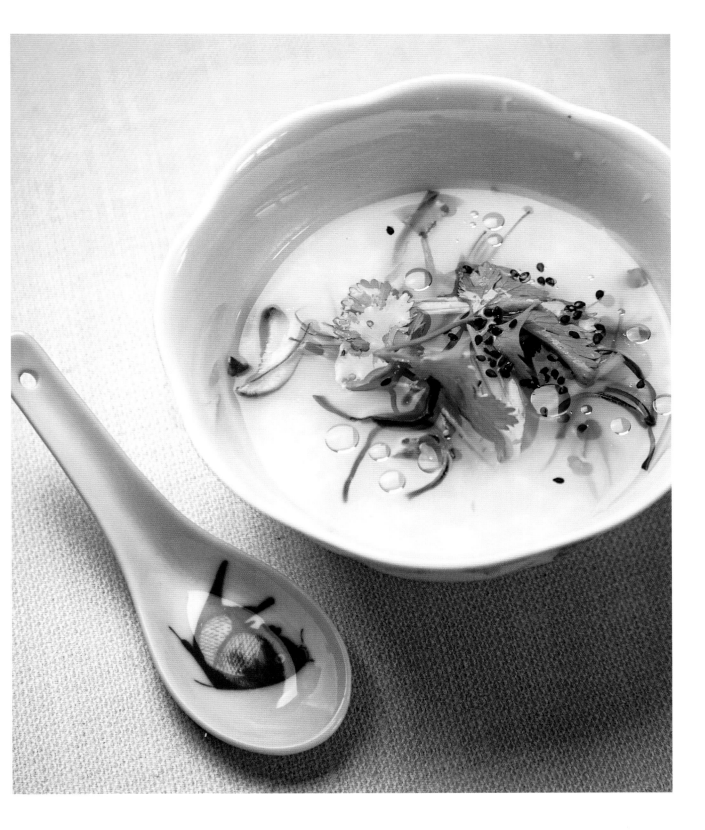

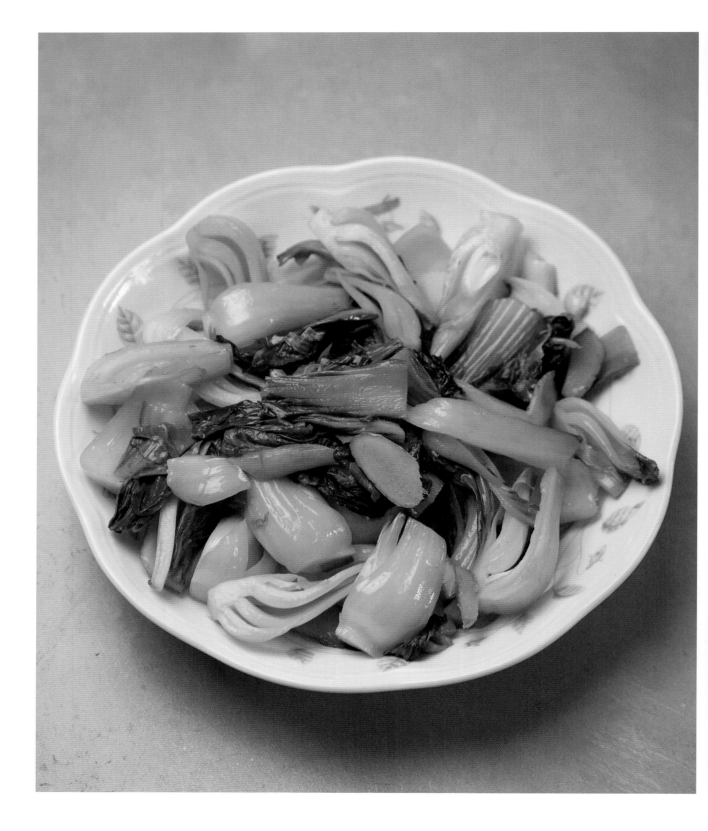

My Special Sauté for Vegetables

In TCM, we tend to avoid raw foods, salads and "cold" foods. I get many questions asking "Why?" and "Don't raw foods contain the most nutrients?"

One essential way to help digestion and your overall health is through a consistent intake of easily digestible and nutritious foods. Cooked foods are much easier to digest than cold or raw foods because they require less Qi (vital energy) to be used in their breakdown. A common misconception is that cooking your vegetables results in losing nutrients. I say that it is better to focus on strengthening the Stomach to be able to absorb nutrients than eating what cannot be absorbed at all. Also, gently cooking your vegetables for a few minutes keeps the nutrition intact.

A light sauté, steam or grill is all vegetables need to be broken down more efficiently by the body while keeping their essence and nutrition intact. Here's how I do it.

Makes 1 serving

3 cloves garlic, sliced

¼ cup (24 g) ginger, sliced

Vegetable of your choice: broccoli, string beans, bok choy, cauliflower or kale

1–5 tbsp (15–75 ml) water (vegetables like broccoli and string beans require more water, bok choy only needs 1 tbsp [15 ml])

High-quality olive oil, to taste

High-quality salt, to taste

Heat your pan over high heat, so it is very hot. You can test it with a droplet of water, making sure it steams when you add the drop! Pan-wise, I like using stainless steel or cast-iron pans. Once the pan is steaming hot, add in the garlic and ginger. Cook for about 30 seconds until fragrant and move them around so they don't burn. Add in your vegetable of choice and mix them around for a few seconds. Add the water in to create steam and cover for 10 to 30 seconds, depending on the vegetable. For example, bok choy needs about 10 seconds covered, while broccoli needs about 2 minutes covered.

Depending on the vegetables, cook for another 1 to 3 minutes and check for color. For example, a green vegetable should look vibrant green, not dark green, and should be crunchy. Transfer the vegetables to a plate and drizzle with olive oil and salt to taste.

Rice Water

Rice water has been used for thousands of years in Asian cultures and cultures around the world. It contains amino acids, vitamins B and E, essential minerals and antioxidants, and can provide healing support to the body in a multitude of ways. It is very beneficial to skin health. Rice contains the antioxidant ferulic acid, as well as an organic compound called allantoin, which helps soothe and heal dry skin, large pores and eczema. To use on skin, place a small amount of rice water on a cotton ball and gently smooth it over your face and neck as a toner. To clean with it, massage it into your skin. Rice water also helps with Lung recovery when recovering from viral infections and boosts the energy of the Spleen to strengthen and support digestion.

Makes about 6–8 cups (1.5–2 quarts)

¾ cup (150 g) uncooked organic white rice
8–10 cups (2–2.5 quarts) filtered water

Rinse the rice. Add the rice and water to a large pot and bring it to a gentle simmer over low to medium heat. Boil the rice until you see the rice kernels open, which usually takes 45 to 60 minutes.

Strain the rice from the water. This will yield several cups of rice water, which you can drink warmed up or at room temperature. It is best to consume on the same day, but you can store it in the fridge and use it within 24 hours for the best results.

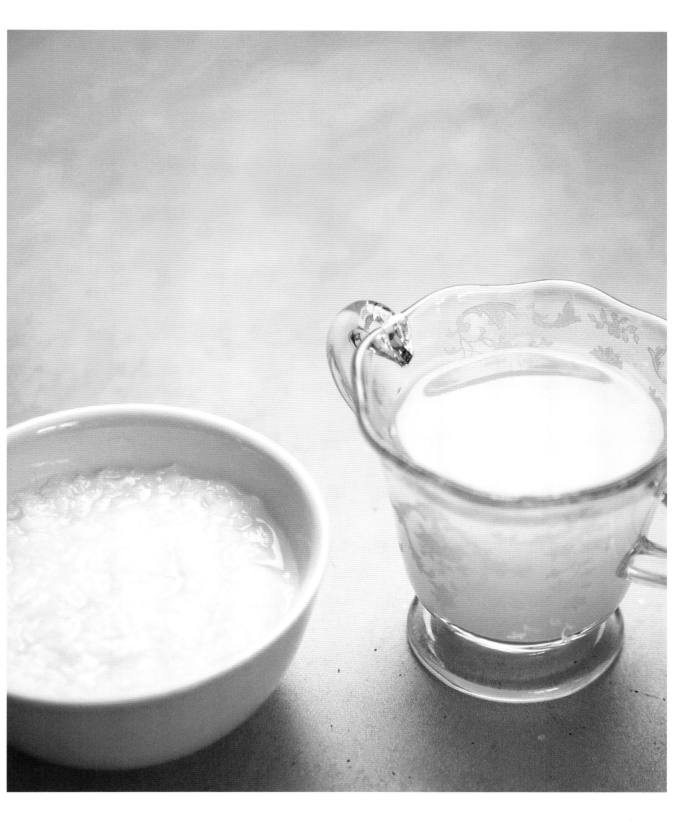

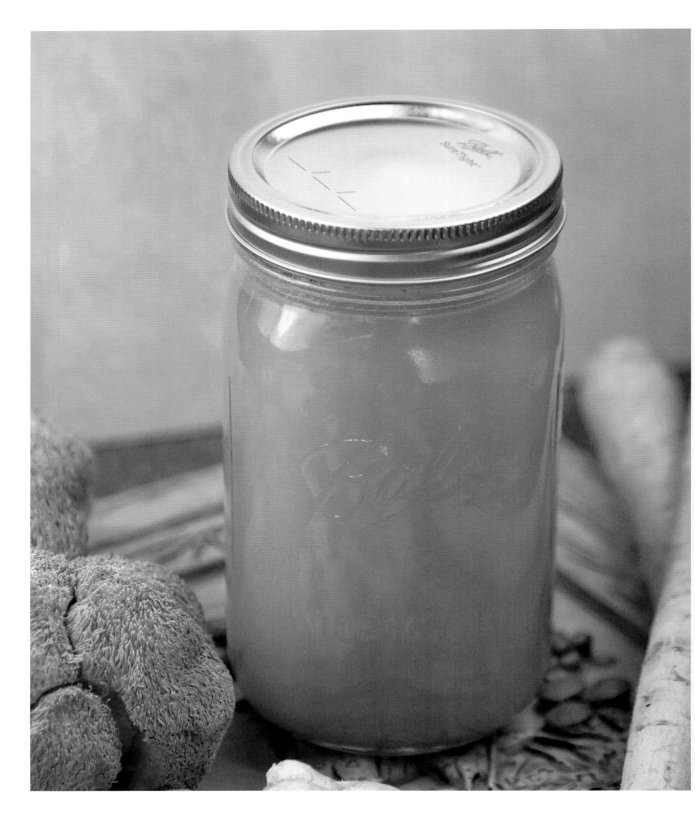

Bone Broths

Beef Bone Broth

Beef Bone Broth is a wonderful way to use up the leftover vegetables and scraps from your fridge. Use herbs, ends and scraps of vegetables, spices and bones in one healing formula. When we consume Bone Broth, we are absorbing the deepest digestible elements available to us, nourishing our body's bones, joints, Blood-building marrow, Kidneys, reproductive system and brain.

Makes 8–12 cups (1.9–2.8 L)

4–5 lb (1.8–2.3 kg) grass-fed beef bones

3 carrots

2 onions

5 celery ribs

2–3 bay leaves

1 tbsp (12 g) peppercorns

Preheat the oven to 350°F (177°C). Roast the beef bones for 30 to 60 minutes, turning them halfway through.

Add the roasted bones to a large pot and add enough filtered water to cover the bones. Separately, use warm water and scrape all the bits off of the roasting pan and add that to the pot. Add in the carrots, onions, celery, bay leaves and peppercorns. You can add whatever other vegetables you like too!

Over medium heat, bring the mixture to a boil, then turn it down to low and simmer for 12 to 24 hours, skimming off what surfaces at the top. Let cool and skim off the fat on top. You can use that for cooking later!

Remove the solid ingredients by straining the broth into mason jars, and store the jars in your fridge or freezer. This will last up to 3 days in the fridge and 6 months in the freezer.

Chicken Bone Broth

Bone Broth is one of the most healing foods to consume. In Chinese medicine, Bone Broth is used because it gifts us the deepest digestible elements available, nourishing our body's bones, joints, Blood-building marrow, Kidneys, reproductive system and brain. In Western medicine, this correlates to the abundance of amino acids it provides, the ability to heal and seal the gut lining and reduce overgrowth of harmful microbes.

Makes 8–12 cups (1.9–2.8 L)

⅛ *cup (12 g) ginger, sliced*
Bones or carcass of a whole chicken
Herbs of choice

Use a deep pot and fill it up three-quarters of the way with filtered water. Add the ginger slices and bring to a boil. Add the bones to the boiling water carefully. Boil for 5 minutes and drain the water, keeping the ginger in the pot. This is how I "clean" the bones. I use the first boil to remove any scum. You can also do this with a fine mesh strainer and just skim the top of the water and not drain it.

If you did drain all the water, add filtered water back to the pot, covering the bones by several inches. Bring the water to a boil. Add in your herbs. Once boiling, cover the pot and simmer for about 1 hour. You can cook longer if you'd like to for a more concentrated, intense flavor. Once finished, sip on it like tea or use it as the base for some yummy noodles! Store the broth in mason jars in the fridge or freezer. This will last up to 3 days in the fridge and 6 months in the freezer.

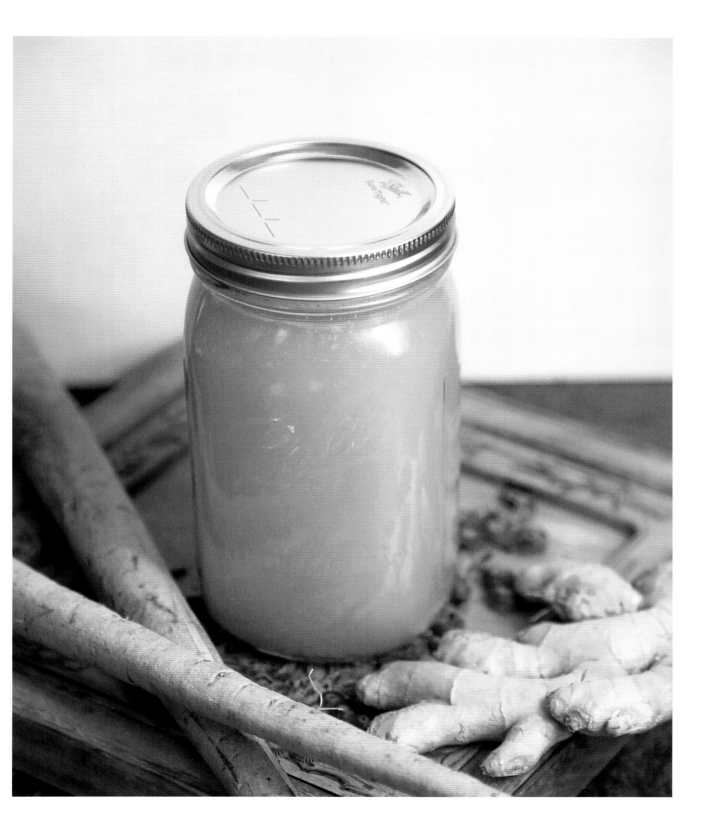

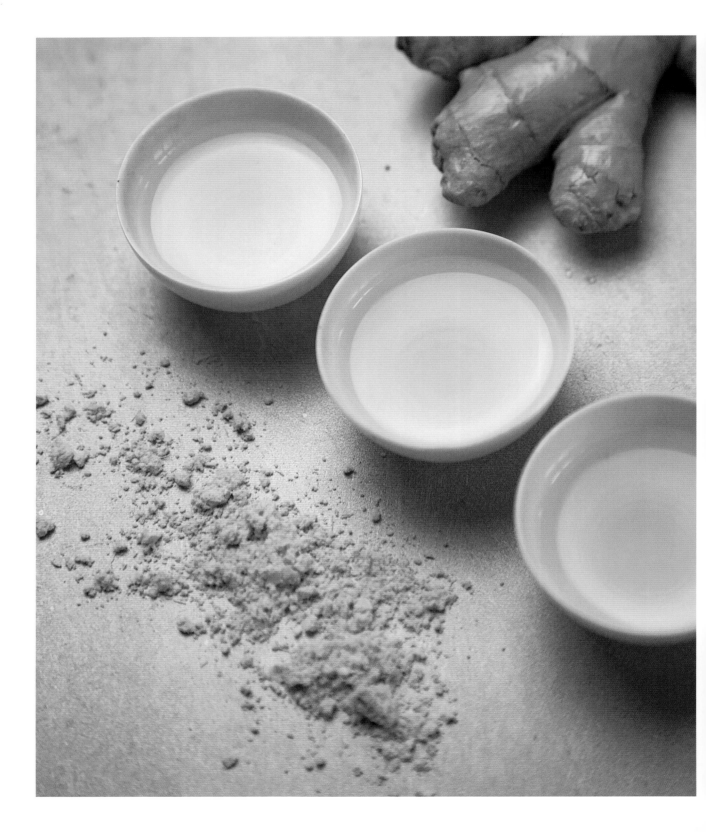

Healing Teas

Dr. Lily's Famous Ginger Power Tea

Ginger Power Tea is the way to get the most potent dehydrated ginger (page 132) into your cup! I'd recommend buying Ginger Power from my website (lilychoinaturalhealing.com), as it is the most potent form and is what I reference continually in the book. I make it myself and it is an organic and pure dehydrated ginger powder. If you're on the go and in a rush, you can swap out Ginger Power for ½ dropper of my Ginger Extract (page 132) in hot water or steep the Ginger Power in hot water for 5 minutes before drinking. And, in a pinch, you can simply use fresh ginger root tea!

Makes 1 serving

If Using Ginger Power

1 cup (240 ml) filtered water
⅛–½ tsp Ginger Power
Honey to taste, optional

Bring the water and Ginger Power to a boil. Boil for 2 minutes on medium-high heat. Pour your tea into a cup. You can use a fine mesh strainer if you don't want the small bits of ginger. Add honey to taste, if desired.

If Using Fresh Ginger

1 cup (240 ml) filtered water
¼ cup (24 g) fresh organic ginger root, smashed
Honey to taste, optional

Bring the water and ginger to a boil. Boil for 10 to 15 minutes on medium heat. The longer you boil the ginger, the stronger the tea will be. Pour your tea into a cup. Add honey to taste, if desired, and enjoy. You can discard the ginger root or use it again.

Booster and Builder Tea

This tea provides us with the ultimate warming essence and can be had all year round. The ginger and Chinese brown sugar strengthen digestion and the red dates tonify Blood.

Makes 1 serving

2 cups (480 ml) filtered water

⅛ cup (12 g) thinly sliced or smashed fresh ginger or ⅛–½ tsp Ginger Power (page 132)

⅛ cup (10 g) red dates, pitted

Chinese brown/black sugar or honey, to taste

Add the water to a small pot along with the ginger and dates. Cover and bring to a boil. Once boiling, reduce the heat and simmer for 15 minutes.

Add the Chinese brown sugar (if using honey, just skip this step—you'll wait to add the honey later). Cover and simmer for another 5 minutes.

Strain the tea into a mug. If using honey, add it now. Let the tea cool to a drinkable temperature. The goal is to drink it while it is still hot for maximum healing!

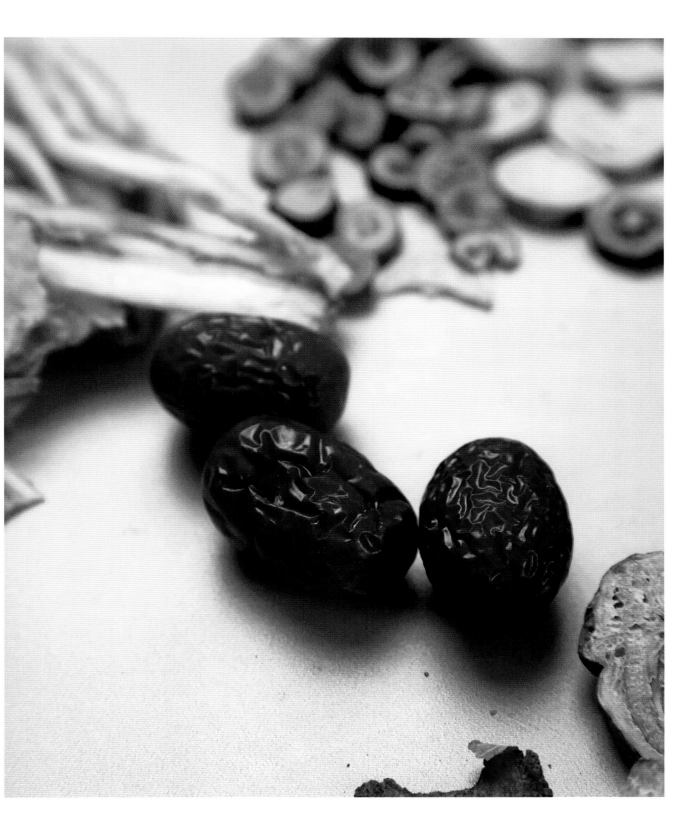

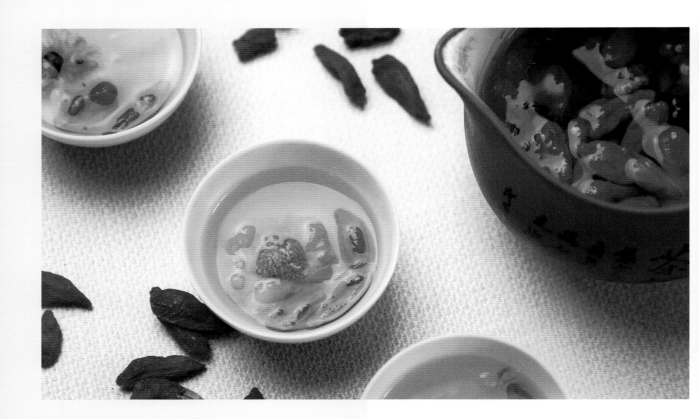

Calming and Cooling Tea

Chrysanthemum is a wonderful flower, which promotes energy, detoxifies the body and skin, and promotes healthy weight and clear vision. You can purchase it online or at your local Asian market. "清肝明目，增強免疫力" is a Chinese saying that means "Chrysanthemum and goji berry clear Liver heat, brighten eyes and increase immunity."

Makes 1 serving

5–9 chrysanthemum flowers
Handful of dried goji berries
2 cups (480 ml) hot filtered water

Cover the chrysanthemums and goji berries with the hot water and steep for 10 minutes. Eat the flowers and goji berries if you like for added benefits, but you don't have to. Drink this once daily.

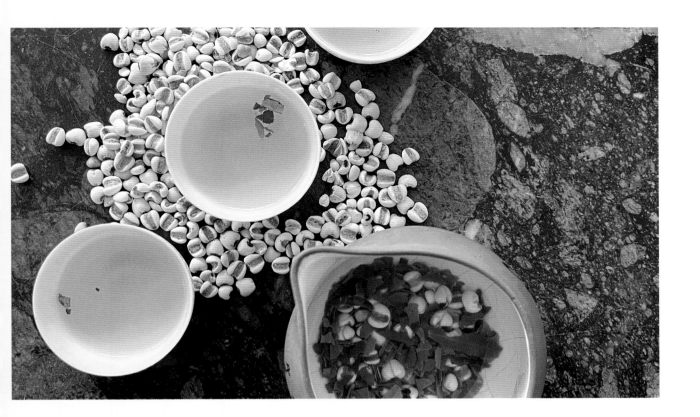

Light as a Feather Tea

As the weather transitions into summer, if you experience a lowered appetite, fatigue and have a general feeling of heaviness, this tea can help! Drink this tea in the warmer months to feel lighter and more energized.

Job's tear (薏仁 Yi Ren), also known as pearl barley, is one of the most effective ways to remove dampness (page 47) from the body. Job's tear also strengthens the Spleen, reduces puffiness and treats edema. Green tea leaves help metabolic function, brain function and contain many antioxidants and bioactive compounds. Do keep in mind that green tea contains caffeine!

Makes 1 serving

¼ cup (50 g) or a handful of uncooked Job's tear
1½ tsp (3–5 g) green tea leaves
2 cups (480 ml) hot filtered water

Roast the Job's tear in a cast-iron or stainless steel pan over low heat until slightly golden brown. Place the Job's tear and green tea leaves in a cup, add the hot water, cover and steep for 10 minutes.

Drink this tea after a meal, not on an empty stomach and not at nighttime as green tea contains caffeine.

Herbal Formulas

Astragalus

Botanical Name: *Milkvetch roots*

Organs and Systems: *Spleen, Lungs, Immunity, Blood Tonic*

Astragalus (黄芪 Huang Qi) has been used for thousands of years in TCM as one of the fifty most fundamental herbs. Apart from using this herb as medicine or in herbal formulas, it is regularly used in soups and various dishes because of its multifunctional "tonifying" ability. In TCM, when we talk about an herb or a food that has the ability to tonify, it means that it contains nourishing, supplementing and strengthening abilities.

Astragalus boosts vital Qi—the life force and vital energy that sustains us. It increases the immunity of the entire body and helps protect it against pathogens like viruses and bacteria.

Astragalus contains a very special compound called cycloastragenol, which has the ability to activate the enzyme telomerase, which, in turn, protects DNA from degradation during replication. This prevents shortening of DNA that specifically helps against disease and aging by extending human life. Polysaccharides and saponins are credited with many of the health benefits provided by the herb.

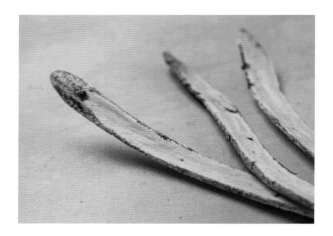

A proprietary extract of the dried root of Astragalus membranaceus, called TA-65, was associated with a significant age-reversal effect in the immune system.[1]

Medicinal Uses of Astragalus

Astragalus plays an important role in preventing and treating diseases such as aplastic anemia, cancer, genital herpes, congestive heart failure, Kidney disease, lupus, oral herpes, flu and respiratory infections, coughing, wheezing, shortness of breath, dizziness, vertigo, spontaneous sweating, palpitations, insomnia, low energy, sallow face and no desire to speak, stress, hormonal imbalance, pale face, fatigue, tired extremities, diarrhea and bruising easily.

---

1   Liu, Ping et al. "Anti-Aging Implications of *Astragalus Membranaceus* (Huangqi): A Well-Known Chinese Tonic." *Aging and disease* vol. 8,6 868-886. 1 Dec. 2017, doi:10.14336/AD.2017.0816.

Du Zhong

Botanical Name: *Eucommia bark*

Organs and Systems: *Musculoskeletal, Tendons, Kidney, Liver*

Du Zhong (杜仲), commonly called rubber tree, originated in central China. The Chinese name for the herb is based on an ancient proverb: "At one time, there was a man named Du Zhong who took this herb and became enlightened; therefore, it was named after him." The part of the tree cultivated and used in TCM is the trunk bark, which is gathered by stripping the bark off the tree in large segments.

This herb activates the Liver and the Kidney systems and helps symptoms that arise from deficiencies in those organs.

Because of its relationship with the Kidney, Du Zhong is a powerhouse antiaging herb—preventing wrinkles, helping weak backs and legs, preventing bone loss and muscle weakness and warming cold hands and feet.

Containing eight different kinds of amino acids, it's also rich in minerals such as zinc, magnesium, potassium, calcium, phosphorous, iron and copper.

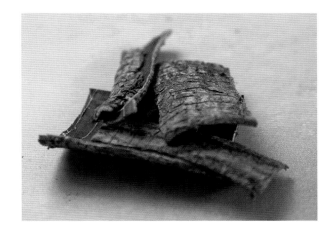

Medicinal Uses of Du Zhong

Du Zhong strengthens our will; lowers cholesterol; promotes natural detoxification; boosts Qi and helps treat fatigue; strengthens knees, bones and sinews; helps treat dizziness that can result from Liver Yang rising, also known as hypertension; and treats metabolic disorders that include diabetes (and its precursor, insulin resistance), Kidney disorders, obesity and cognitive decline.

Ginger

Botanical Name: *Zingiber officinale*

Organs and Systems: *Spleen, Stomach, Liver, Kidney, Lung*

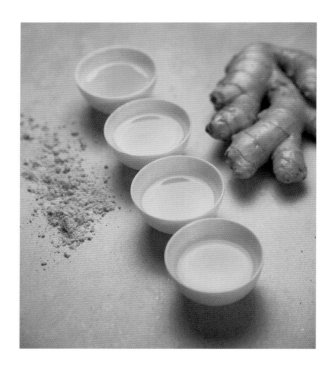

Ginger (薑) is the most warming food we can consume and you can have it raw, cooked, dehydrated, dried and even candied!

Ginger is an antioxidant, and an anti-inflammatory, anti-cancer, anti-proliferation, anti-invasion and natural antibiotic herb. Therefore, it is a great resource for our precious Yang energy and total body wellness.

Ginger Power is my dehydrated organic ginger powder that I make through a process of turning dehydrated ginger into a powder form. This is not the same as buying ground ginger from your local supermarket, however. It is a labor of love to create the freshest and most potent ginger available. Ginger Extract is my liquid version of the powder form. Both are available on my website (lilychoinatural-healing.com).

Dehydrated ginger provides antioxidant, antimicrobial, antibacterial and anti-inflammatory support. It helps in the treatment of cancer, hypertension, diabetes, excess weight, digestive disorders and the common cold.

Medicinal Uses of Ginger Power

Ginger Power helps with nauseous sensations and stomach discomfort, chronic headaches and migraines, acid reflux, viral and bacterial infections in the stomach and mouth, joint pain, dampness removal, fatigue, cold hands and feet and premenstrual syndrome. It also assists in the removal of mold, parasites and toxins.

Goji Berries

Botanical Name: *Lycium*

Organs and Systems: *Liver, Lung, Blood*

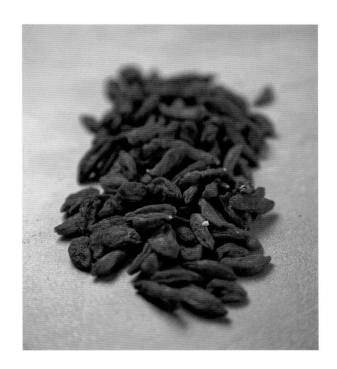

Goji berries (枸杞子 Gou Qi Zi) have been used for thousands of years as both food and medicine. My mentor, who still practices medicine at 97 years old, swears by consuming them daily.

Because of their neutral nature, they are extremely versatile and can be used by those with either a Yin or Yang deficiency. These berries can improve neurological and psychological performance and gastrointestinal functions. They also increase beneficial bacteria in the gut, making them probiotics. Goji berries help treat many Stomach conditions, including colitis, and offer antioxidant support by way of alleviating oxidative stress.

The eyes love this berry! Because of the amount of time the average person spends in front of a screen, it should be especially noted how much they help the eyes. Goji berries contain a high amount of taurine, an amino acid which is a building block of human proteins found in the brain, spinal cord, heart and muscle cells, skeletal muscle tissue and retinas. Taurine has antioxidant, anti-inflammatory and immuno-modulating properties that can protect the retina. Goji berries excel at providing eye support as a result of diabetes complications, macular degeneration, floaters, poor eyesight, cataracts, blurred vision, eye twitching, red eyes and glaucoma.

Medicinal Uses of Goji Berries

Goji berries aid in patterns of Yin and Blood deficiency, lower back pain, nocturnal emissions, eye conditions caused by Kidney or Liver deficiency, dizziness, blurred vision, cancer, lower cholesterol, fatigue, stamina, low back or knee pain, building energy, balancing blood sugar, longevity, glaucoma, skin irritations and diseases, enhancing immune function, supporting liver function, anxiety, depression, stress, dry coughing, cognitive function, male infertility and hypertension.

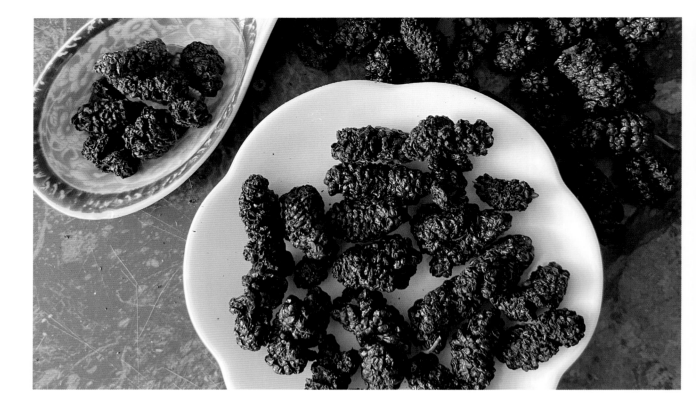

Mulberries

Botanical Name: *Morus*

Organs and Systems: *Blood, Kidneys, Digestive*

Mulberries (桑葚子 Sang Shen Zi) contain anti-oxidant, anti-inflammatory, anti-tumor and anti-diabetic effects, as well as cardiovascular and hepato- and neuroprotective properties.[1]

Studies have shown that mulberry fruits possess several potential pharmacological health benefits, including anti-cholesterol, anti-obesity and hepato-protective effects.[2]

Medicinal Uses of Mulberries

Mulberries tonify the Blood, lubricate intestines and nourish Yin and body fluid. They also help with hot flashes, fatigue, night sweats, vaginal dryness, lower back soreness, discomfort or weakness, dizziness, tinnitus, constipation, dry skin, unquenchable thirst, irritability, insomnia, quelling anger and frustration, nocturnal emissions, sore throat, chronic swelling of gums and chronic toothaches.

1   Huang Hui-Pei et al., "Mulberry (sang shèn zi) and its bioactive compounds, the chemoprevention effects and molecular mechanisms in vitro and in vivo," *Journal of Traditional and Complementary Medicine* 3, no. 1 (2013): 7-15, 10.4103/2225-4110.106535

2   Zhang Hongxia et al., "Effects of Mulberry Fruit (Morus alba L.) Consumption on Health Outcomes: A Mini-Review," *Antioxidants (Basel, Switzerland)* 7, no. (2018): 69, 10.3390/antiox7050069

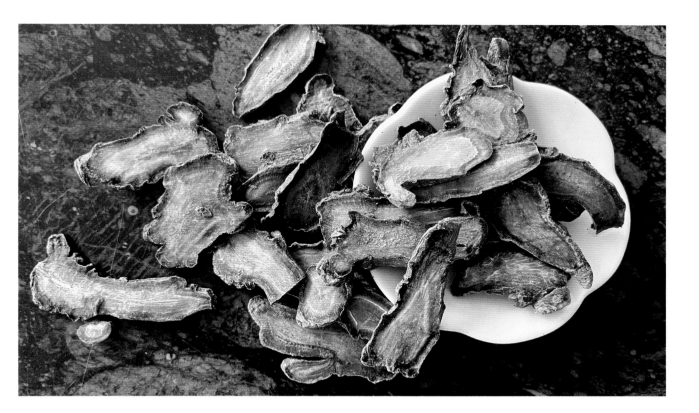

San Qi

Botanical Name: *Panax notoginseng*

Organs and Systems: *Cardiovascular, Nervous*

舒根活胳 is a Chinese saying for San Qi that means "soothes the tendons and activates the meridians."

San Qi (三七) is a powerful adaptogen with anti-inflammatory and anti-apoptotic properties, meaning it prevents apoptosis or the death of cells. This herb can regenerate cells and protect the mitochondria—the structures within cells that produce energy. When mitochondria are compromised, the metabolism experiences dysfunction at varying levels. These energy producers are quite sensitive. Symptoms like fatigue, premature aging, memory loss and pain (among many more) manifest when they are damaged.

In Latin, the word "panax" means "cure-all." Known for its ability to treat all Blood disorders, San Qi rose to notoriety during the Qing dynasty. Famous herbalist Li Shizhen referred to it as Jin Bu Huan (Not Even Exchanged for Gold) and some later herb primers went so far as to call it "the king of all herbs"—a status it has maintained until today.

Medicinal Uses of San Qi

San Qi treats bleeding of nearly any external trauma or internal disharmony, pain and swelling from trauma or arthritis, chest pain, abdominal pain, traumatic swelling, joint pain, stress-related disorders, mood disorders and depression.

Schisandra

Botanical Name: *Schisandra chinensis*

Organs and Systems: *Immunity, Nervous, Endocrine*

Schisandra (五味子) was written about in China's first herbal dictionary in the first century BC. It was described as a superior and elite herb to be used daily to promote longevity and well-being, something I still find true to this day. The power of this berry lies in the fact that it features all five of the taste senses at once, each denoting its own medicinal application.

Sweet: for the Spleen, restores energy and immune system function

Salty: for the Kidneys, provides minerals and nourishes the Blood

Sour: for the Liver, detoxes and promotes digestion

Bitter: for the Heart, stimulates digestion, treats inflammation and detoxes

Pungent: strengthens organs, stimulates Blood circulation and is especially beneficial to the Lungs and Large Intestine

One of schisandra's greatest attributes is its ability to cleanse the Liver, due in part to its strong antioxidant content. It works by aiding in the detoxification process of binding to waste and toxins and eliminating them from the body. It then stimulates the growth of new liver cells and shields the Liver from toxins. Schisandra is also considered an adaptogen. It addresses the adrenals and responds to excess stress by modulating endocrine and immune functions. Schisandra combats poor metabolism symptoms such as fatigue, poor endurance and blood sugar swings. It also helps with emotional stress and stress from overworking by tonifying the adrenal cortex and the Liver.

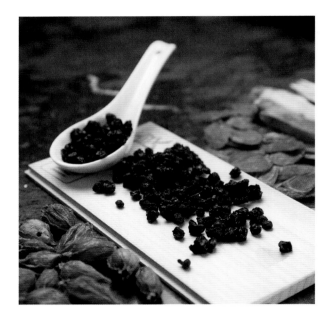

Schisandra has always been popular in China, especially among the wealthy class, to promote beautiful skin and provide protection from sun and wind damage. Even in ancient times, in one painting, Magu, the goddess of beauty and eternal youth, is pictured serving a tray of schisandra, reishi (considered the herb of immortality) and a "peach of longevity" to her immortal friends. Because of the astringent nature of schisandra, it helps the skin hold moisture to keep it glowing, plump and supple.

Medicinal Uses of Schisandra

Schisandra helps with patterns of Lung and Kidney deficiency, adrenal fatigue, chronic hepatitis C, chronic coughs, nocturnal emissions, spermatorrhea, vaginal discharge, frequent urination, premature aging, excessive sweating with thirst or dry throat, night sweats, irritability, palpitations, premenstrual syndrome, chronic diarrhea, fatty liver, erectile dysfunction, exhaustion, memory loss, lower cholesterol, pneumonia, dysentery, chemo-protective, immunity boosting, dream-disturbed sleep and insomnia due to injury to Heart and Kidney Yin.

Self-Heal

Botanical Name: *Prunella vulgaris*

Organs and Systems: *Liver*

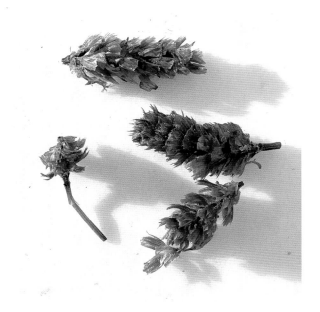

Self-Heal (夏枯草 Xia Ku Cao) is an ancient herb of significant medicinal importance. It possesses anti-inflammatory, anti-diabetic and anti-cancer properties, as well as regulating immune function capabilities.[1]

In TCM, it is classified as clearing heat and purging fire and considered to have its primary effect on the syndrome of Liver Yang Rising, which is a common pattern in our modern world. Liver Yang Rising is caused by stress, alcohol, excess caffeine, emotional imbalances like intense anger or frustration, lack of sleep and a poor diet. These lifestyle habits create a fire that rises in the body, usually exposing itself through symptoms in the upper body.

You can utilize this herb by steeping it in dried form as tea or using the extract version in tincture form, available on my website (lilychoinaturalhealing.com).

Medicinal Uses of Self-Heal

Self-Heal aids acne, irritability, outbursts of anger, constipation, dream-disturbed sleep, painful red eyes, sore eyeballs at night, headaches, dizziness, acute mastitis, goiter and hypertension.

---

1   Mir Reyaz Hassan et al., "Prunella vulgaris L: Critical Pharmacological, Expository Traditional Uses and Extensive Phytochemistry: A Review," *Current Drug Discovery Technologies* 19, no. 1 (2022): 10.2174/1570163818666621020318 1542

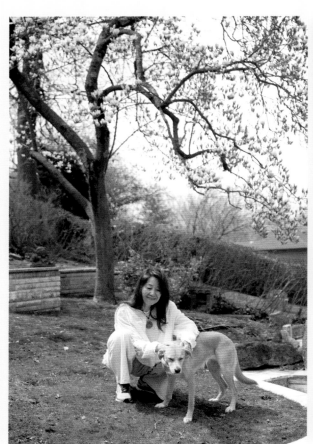 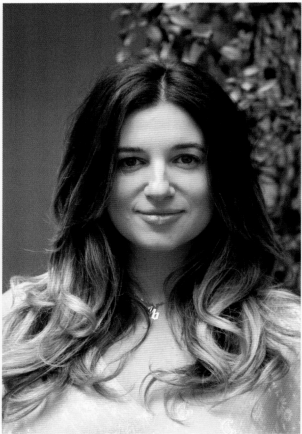

Acknowledgments

Dr. Lily Choi

I would like to thank my mom and my dad for their inspiration, joy and care. I thank them for being the best role models for me.

About the Authors

Dr. Lily Choi

Dr. Lily Choi is a licensed acupuncturist (L.Ac) best known for her bustling practice in New York City, Lily Choi Natural Healing, where she treats thousands of patients with traditional Chinese medicine practices. Lily employs Master Tung's acupuncture system along with traditional Chinese acupuncture methods in her patient care. She was first introduced to Master Tung's system when she lived in Hong Kong, China. He is referred to as the greatest acupuncture master who ever lived. She received her master's in acupuncture from the New York College of Traditional Chinese Medicine after immigrating to the United States, as well as her doctor of acupuncture (D.Ac) from the Pacific College of Oriental Medicine. Lily is board-certified by the National Certification Commission for Acupuncture and Oriental Medicine in acupuncture.

Lily also runs popular Instagram and TikTok accounts where she shares her knowledge of TCM with followers all over the world. You can keep up with her journey @lilychoinaturalhealing. You can also check out her website for further resources and browse the tinctures, herbal and skin care products, and authentic jade gua sha tool she handmakes and sells at lilychoinaturalhealing.com.

Lily's real passion, just like her dad, is her herbal formulas and creating her own concoctions along with traditional formulas. The process, she says, "brings her great contentment."

Bess Koutroumanis

Bess Koutroumanis worked in the fashion industry in New York City for twelve years until she couldn't ignore the feeling of being called to help others. Through her own journey of healing the body and mind, she became passionate about helping others with similar methods. Bess lives by the principles of TCM but within the modern world. She has been Dr. Lily's apprentice for more than four years.

Bess is also a multimedia artist with an emphasis on helping people heal through her art and words. She lives in Los Angeles, California, and seeks solace in nature and connecting with the elements.

Index